Billing and Collecting for Your Mental Health Practice

D1737388

Billing and Collecting for Your Mental Health Practice

Effective Strategies and Ethical Practice

Jeffrey E. Barnett

Steven Walfish

American Psychological Association

Washington, DC

Published by
American Psychological Association
750 First Street, NE
Washington, DC 20002
www.apa.org

To order
APA Order Department
P.O. Box 92984
Washington, DC 20090-2984
Tel: (800) 374-2721; Direct: (202) 336-5510
Fax: (202) 336-5502; TDD/TTY: (202) 336-6123
Online: www.apa.org/pubs/books
E-mail: order@apa.org

In the U.K., Europe, Africa, and the Middle East, copies may be ordered from
American Psychological Association
3 Henrietta Street
Covent Garden, London
WC2E 8LU England

Typeset in Meridien by Circle Graphics, Inc., Columbia, MD

Printer: Edwards Brothers, Inc., Ann Arbor, MI
Cover Designer: Minker Design, Sarasota, FL

The opinions and statements published are the responsibility of the authors, and such opinions and statements do not necessarily represent the policies of the American Psychological Association.

Library of Congress Cataloging-in-Publication Data

Barnett, Jeffrey E.
  Billing and collecting for your mental health practice : effective strategies and ethical practice/by Jeffrey E. Barnett and Steven Walfish. — 1st ed.
      p. ; cm.
  Includes bibliographical references.
  ISBN-13: 978-1-4338-1017-6
  ISBN-10: 1-4338-1017-4
  1. Mental health services—Practice. 2. Mental health services—Administration. 3. Mental health services—Finance. 4. Medical ethics. I. Walfish, Steven. II. American Psychological Association. III. Title.

  [DNLM: 1. Mental Health Services—organization & administration. 2. Practice Management, Medical—economics. 3. Financial Management—methods. 4. Private Practice—ethics. 5. Private Practice organization & administration. WM 30]

  RA790.75.B37 2012
  362.196'890068—dc22
                                        2011002432

British Library Cataloguing-in-Publication Data
A CIP record is available from the British Library.

Printed in the United States of America
First Edition

DOI: 10.1037/13017-000

Contents

8

Fraud, Abuse, and Case Examples 87

Billing and Collecting for Your Mental Health Practice

Introduction 1

Although mental health clinicians receive extensive training in the clinical aspects of their professional roles, they typically receive minimal, if any, education and training in the business aspects of private practice. After completing their clinical training and entering practice, clinicians will want to be compensated for the clinical services they provide. If all clients paid cash for the services provided at the end of each session, little additional assistance would be necessary. However, because many clinicians work with clients who use their health care insurance to provide reimbursement for services provided, professionals must be well versed in billing and the collection of fees. This training must include practical aspects of how to bill for services rendered and how to collect fees owed, along with how to do so ethically and legally.

We have provided a brief, readable, practical, and user-friendly book that fills this void in most clinicians' training. This practical book should be of interest and value to all clinicians who bill for their services through third parties, such as managed care companies and health insurance companies. Furthermore, even those clinicians who are out-of-network providers and those who work on a fee-for-service basis will benefit from many aspects of this book because they must collect fees, even if directly from their clients.

This book provides specific and practical guidance on the technical aspects of billing. We discuss how to bill when a client is paying for services directly, how to bill accurately and ethically when a client chooses to use insurance, and how to optimize collections regarding collection of co-pays and using credit cards. Our emphasis is placed on the ethical framework that guides all decisions regarding billing and collecting. We place the focus on protecting clients' rights in the billing and collections processes, outline steps for providing clients with informed consent about billing practices and procedures, and discuss other issues relevant to ethical and legal practice in billing and collecting fees.

Everyone intends to be ethical and remain within the bounds of the law. However, not everyone succeeds in this regard, through either acts of omission or of commission. This is not a book on bookkeeping and accounting. Rather, we intend it as resource for those in private mental health practice to assist them with effectively and ethically billing and collecting for the services they provide. We have collectively been in practice for more than 50 years and have grappled with concerns regarding billing and collecting in an effective and ethical manner since day one. It is our hope that through the presentation of conceptual issues and practical examples of what we and our colleagues have encountered in private practice, our readers will increase their collections and reduce the likelihood of an ethical or legal transgression.

The book is organized into six primary chapters. Chapter 2 outlines ethical considerations in the billing and collection process. Issues related to setting fees, anticipating clients' financial limitations, making financial arrangements, raising fees responding to clients who do not pay their fees, handling referrals and fees, and billing in an accurate and nonfraudulent manner are discussed. Chapter 3 focuses on the importance of the written financial agreement between clinician and client that is established at the beginning of treatment as part of the informed-consent agreement. We identify impediments on the part of both the client and clinician that may interfere with billing and collecting, along with ways to overcome these impediments. Chapter 4 focuses on how clinicians actually get reimbursed for their services. We discuss payment when clients are paying out of pocket for services or using their insurance company to pay for part or all of their treatment. This includes accurate billing of the insurance company, collection of co-pays due from the client, acceptance of credit card payments, and special billing circumstances that may apply with Medicare and workers compensation claims. Chapter 5 focuses on the advantages and disadvantages of using a billing service versus doing all of the billing and collecting on your own. This decision is based not only on the practicality and costs of billing and collecting but also on the personal values and personality of the clinician. Chapter 6 focuses on billing in the forensic area of practice. This includes discussion of fee setting, what the clinician is paid to do, when to get paid, and the need to avoid contingency payment arrangements in personal injury cases. Chapter 7 discusses the most common causes of inaccurate billing and the most common types of ethical dilemmas clinicians face in the billing process. Finally, Chapter 8 discusses the difference between fraud and abuse, provides illustrative case examples, and offers suggestions for how to prevent their occurrence.

We thank Linda McCarter, our acquisitions editor at APA Books. Her input helped shape the presentation of our ideas, and we believe the book is stronger because of her wisdom. We also appreciate the work of Beth Hatch, our development editor at APA Books, who helped to improve the manuscript.

We welcome feedback, comments, and questions from our readers. Please do not hesitate to contact Jeff Barnett (drjbarnett1@verizon.net) or Steve Walfish (psychpubs@aol.com).

The Ethics of Billing, Collecting, and Financial Arrangements
A Working Framework for Clinicians

2

The reality of being in private practice is that our clients pay our salaries. It is only by generating fees and effectively collecting them that we can keep our practices viable. Yet our attempts to maximize profits occur in the context of a therapeutic relationship. How we balance the business and clinical aspects of our practice in an ethical manner is an essential concern for all clinicians.

A focus on ethical practice is a hallmark of our work, and the ethics codes of each of the mental health professions are built on a group of underlying principles (Beauchamp & Childress, 1994; Kitchener, 1984) that provide guidance in all areas of professional practice. These underlying ethical principles include the following:

- Beneficence: To help those we serve and to be guided by their best interests in all we do.
- Nonmaleficence: To avoid or prevent exploitation and harm of those we serve.
- Fidelity: Exercising faithfulness in our obligations to others.
- Autonomy: Promoting others' independence of us over time and not creating needless dependence on us.
- Integrity: Being truthful and honest; keeping all agreements and promises made.

▪ Justice: Being fair in all interactions and ensuring equal access to high-quality services for all individuals.

These principles form the basis of the specific ethical standards that comprise each mental health profession's ethics code. Areas of practice typically emphasized in these standards include a comprehensive informed-consent process, as well as competence in clinical practice to include multicultural competence, confidentiality, boundaries and multiple relationships, termination and abandonment, advertising and public statements, media presentations, assessment, research and publishing, supervision, and teaching, among others (see American Counseling Association [ACA], 2005; American Psychological Association [APA], 2010a; National Association of Social Workers [NASW], 1999).

In addition to ethical standards directly relevant to the clinical services that clinicians provide, standards exist that emphasize the business aspects of mental health practice. The Ethical Principles of Psychologists and Code of Conduct (APA Ethics Code; APA, 2010a) addresses these issues in Standards 6.04, Fees and Financial Arrangements; 6.05, Barter With Clients/Patients; 6.06, Accuracy in Reports to Payors and Funding Sources; 6.07, Referrals and Fees; and 6.03, Withholding Records for Nonpayment. Similar standards are found in the American Counseling Association's Code of Ethics (ACA, 2005) to include Standard A.10, Fees and Bartering (which includes Accepting Fees From Agency Clients, Establishing Fees, Nonpayment of Fees, Bartering, and Receiving Gifts), and Standard C.6.b., Reports to Third Parties. Similarly, the NASW Code of Ethics (NASW, 1999) includes Standards 1.13, Payment for Services; 2.06, Referral for Services; 3.05, Billing; 4.04, Dishonesty, Fraud, and Deception; and 4.06, Misrepresentation.

Thus, it is clear that the ethics codes of the mental health professions apply not only to clinical aspects of practice but also to billing, fees, and financial arrangements. Additionally, as will be addressed, specific laws and regulations exist that affect the fee and billing activities of clinicians. Knowledge of ethical standards, laws, and regulations relevant to fees, billing, and financial arrangements is essential for the appropriate and ethical conduct of clinicians.

In this chapter, we discuss several aspects of the billing and collections process as it intersects with ethical practice. These include (a) integrating financial issues into the informed-consent process, (b) understanding informed consent as an ongoing process rather than a solitary event, (c) anticipating financial limitations that may affect clients' ability to pay for services, (d) the role that noninsurance third parties may play in the billing and collections process, (e) how to ethically and appropriately raise fees, (f) how to respond when clients do not pay agreed-on fees, (g) negotiating the use of alternative methods to pay for services, (h) referrals and fees, (i) the need for accurate billing, and (j) how to prevent fraudulent billing.

Overview of Informed Consent

Informed consent is described by Barnett, Wise, Johnson-Greene, and Buckey (2007) as "a shared decision-making process in which the professional communicates sufficient information to the other individual so that she or he may make an informed decision about participation in the professional relationship" (p. 179). Other authors have added to this definition of informed consent, such as Beahrs and Gutheil (2001) who described informed consent as "the process of sharing information with patients that is essential to their ability to make rational choices among multiple options" (p. 4). The fact that various clinicians may have different fees, financial policies, and financial arrangements makes the sharing of this information especially relevant. Failure to do so could be seen as severely limiting the client's ability to make an informed decision about entering treatment with a particular clinician. The fact that third party payors (e.g., insurance companies) are often involved in the payment of some part of the fees on behalf of the client can serve to complicate the financial disclosure process. By sharing sufficient information with clients, they are better able to choose from among the many options available to them for mental health services.

A number of financial matters should be addressed as part of the informed-consent process. These include the discussion of the client's financial limitations as well as an accurate explanation of fees, financial policies and arrangements, charges for various services to be provided, and what reasonably to anticipate with regard to insurance coverage and reimbursement. Furthermore, whether the clinician participates in specific insurance and managed care plans, is an in-network provider for certain insurance companies, or solely follows a fee-for-service model should all be discussed. It is each clinician's responsibility to ensure that clients understand the information presented and their implications with regard to the services the client is seeking (Barnett, Wise, et al., 2007).

When clients are using their health insurance benefits for reimbursement of the fees for services provided, it is important for clinicians to clarify the limits of each client's insurance coverage from the outset. Pomerantz (2005) offered a number of questions clients may have that should be answered during the informed-consent process. These include the following:

- How much does psychotherapy cost?
- Do you accept my insurance?
- How much does my insurance company pay (percentage, total)?
- What forms of payment do you accept (cash, credit cards, check)?
- How often will I need to pay?
- Can fees go up at some point?
- What information will my insurance company be given?
- What information will my employer be given? (p. 355)

Important pieces of information to clarify also include the following:

- Are there any limits to coverage, such as a maximum number of treatment sessions per year?
- Is there a deductible before insurance benefits are paid?
- Are there certain disorders or diagnoses (e.g., parent–child communication problem, learning disabilities, partner-communication problem, obesity) that are not covered?

It is clear that clients will want and need to know what portion of fees charged will be their responsibility and what portion will be covered by their insurance. If this cannot be determined before an initial insurance claim is processed, this fact should be clarified with the client from the outset. Clients will also want to know whether you will file the insurance claim and wait to be reimbursed or whether they must pay for the session up front and wait to be reimbursed by their insurance company. Additionally, it is especially important that clients are informed of one's policy on canceled and missed appointments, because most insurers will only provide reimbursement for services actually rendered. Furthermore, as Knapp and VandeCreek (2008) recommended, fees for all nonclinical services such as letter or report writing and fees for time spent on telephone calls or e-mails, with either clients or collateral contacts, should be fully addressed as well and should comport with contractual obligations with insurers.

Accuracy and honesty in the setting of fees and in how information about them is shared with clients is essential. Standard 6.04(c), Fees and Financial Arrangements, of the APA (2010a) Ethics Code clearly states that "Psychologists do not misrepresent their fees." Similarly, Standard 4.04, Dishonesty, Fraud, and Deception, of the NASW (1999) Code of Ethics states that "Social workers should not participate in, condone, or be associated with dishonesty, fraud, or deception." Thus, all information provided to clients should be presented accurately, both verbally and in a written financial agreement to which the client can refer back over time. The use of a written financial agreement and open discussion during the informed-consent procedure also helps ensure that clients have realistic expectations of the clinician and about treatment from the outset. It is important to minimize the risk of misunderstandings that may have an adverse impact on the professional relationship and the clinical services provided.

Informed Consent as an Ethical Mandate

Snyder and Barnett (2006) emphasized that benefits of the informed-consent process include "promoting client autonomy and self-determination, minimizing the risk of exploitation and harm, fostering rational decision-making, and enhancing the therapeutic alliance" (p. 37). Only by fulfilling our informed-consent obligations with clients can we achieve these goals. Failure to provide clients with the information needed to make an informed decision about participation in the professional relationship, including policies and procedures for billing and collecting fees, can jeopardize each of these goals. This point is well made in a study by Sullivan, Martin, and Handelsman (1993) in which they surveyed potential consumers of mental health services about the use of informed consent. These researchers found that consumers rated those professionals who engaged in an informed-consent process with clients as more expert and trustworthy. Furthermore, these clients would be more likely to refer friends to these professionals and to use the professionals themselves compared with clients with mental health professionals who did not provide informed consent.

The inclusion of fees, financial policies, and financial arrangements in every client's informed-consent agreement is consistent with the dictates of the ethics codes of the mental health professions. The APA (2010a) Ethics Code includes these issues as essential elements required in Standard 10.01, Informed Consent to Therapy. Content that must be addressed in each client's informed-consent agreement include "the nature and course of therapy, *fees,* involvement of third parties, and limits of confidentiality" (emphasis added). Further, in Standard 6.04, Fees and Financial Arrangements, the APA Ethics Code requires that at the earliest time possible, psychologists and those to whom they provide professional services "reach an agreement specifying compensation and billing arrangements."

The NASW (2008) Ethics Code identifies informed consent as essential for helping to promote each client's self-determination (Standard 1.02, Self-Determination). In Standard 1.03, Informed Consent, the NASW

Ethics Code includes "limits to services because of the requirements of a third party payer" and "relevant costs" as essential elements of each client's informed-consent agreement (para. 25). The ACA (2005) Code of Ethics similarly mandates inclusion of fees and billing arrangements in each client's informed consent and requires that "counselors take steps to ensure that clients understand the implications of . . . fees and billing arrangements" (p. 4). Principal 7.2 of the American Association of Marriage and Family Therapists Ethics Code (AAMFT; 2001) states that

> prior to entering into the therapeutic relationship marriage and family therapists clearly disclose and explain to clients all financial arrangements and fees related to professional services, including charges for canceled or missed appointments, use of collection agencies, and the procedure for obtaining payment from the client, if payment is denied by a third party payor. (para. 66)

Thus, it can be seen that there is wide agreement in the ethics codes of the mental health professions that these issues must be openly and thoughtfully addressed in each client's informed consent.

As is true with other important informed-consent issues, fees and financial arrangements should not be discussed on a single occasion but should be reviewed over time throughout the professional relationship (Barnett, Wise, et al., 2007; C. B. Fisher & Oransky, 2008). There are two important reasons to address informed consent from a process model approach (Pomerantz, 2005). First, clients are presented with a significant amount of information that they need to absorb and understand, and when this information is shared at the beginning of the professional relationship, the client is frequently in an emotionally charged state, if not in emotional crisis. The likelihood of clients concentrating on, and fully understanding, the implications of all information shared with them under these circumstances is not great. Second, situations change over the course of treatment. For example, clients' insurance coverage or their ability to afford treatment may change; the clinician may discontinue participation in an insurance network or raise the fees charged. Thus, revisiting informed-consent issues over the course of the professional relationship is viewed as essential for meeting our ethical obligations to clients.

When Should the Informed-Consent Process Begin?

The ethics codes of the mental health professions advise that informed consent be provided as soon as is feasible in the professional relationship. As Pomerantz (2005) has highlighted, this may mean that different issues are discussed at different points in time. However, one should not assume that as early as is feasible begins during the first session with a new client. Instead, it is recommended that informed consent related to financial matters first be addressed even before the initial appointment with clients. Potential clients have the right to know the fees they will be expected to pay, whether insurance is accepted, how payment is expected, and the like before the initial session. Such information is so important to many individuals that it may be a deciding factor whether they will be able to seek the services of a particular clinician.

Referrals to clinicians come from many sources. These may include primary care physicians, other mental health professionals who are colleagues or who may know of the mental health professional by reputation, schools, friends or colleagues of past clients, and others. These referral sources may not be aware of a particular clinician's fees, payment and billing practices, financial policies, or participation in insurance and managed care. Ensuring that every potential referral source in one's local area has such up-to-date information is not likely to be feasible.

Potential clients may be referred to you with every intention of working with you because of a strong personal recommendation received from an individual whose opinions they trust. However, the recommendation about the types of clients you work with and the fine job you did previously are not the only information potential clients will need. Many may be greatly limited by financial restrictions such as the need to work with a clinician who is an in-network provider for their insurance company. Thus, making information about fees and financial policies and arrangements available to potential clients is of great importance (rather than their finding this out during the initial session) and should be seen as the first step in the informed-consent process.

One way to begin sharing information with potential clients to assist them in making informed decisions about with whom to enter treatment is the use of a professional website. In addition to basic information such as your name, degree, licensure status, areas of professional expertise, office location, and *the like*, information on the website can include the following:

- Fees for each type of service provided: Do you charge different fees for the initial evaluation session, for psychotherapy versus psychological testing, for forensic services, etc.?
- How payment is accepted: Do you only accept cash or personal checks? Do you accept credit card payments, and if so, what type?
- When payment is expected: Is payment expected at the beginning of each appointment, at the end of each appointment, monthly? If payment is not expected at each appointment, do you bill the client?

▪ Participation in insurance or managed care: For which insurance and managed care plans are you an in-network provider? Does the potential client need to obtain preauthorization before the first appointment, and if so, how is this done? If you are an out-of-network provider, for which insurance plans does this apply and how does this affect coverage of professional services provided by you for the client?

Thus, sharing information about fees and financial policies and expectations should begin before the first appointment with a new client. This is important because such knowledge could affect the potential client's decision about seeking professional services from you and because of the need for some clients to contact their insurer to obtain preauthorization before the first appointment to have it covered by their insurance. Finding out after the first appointment that it was not covered by the insurer is not a surprise clients will be pleased to receive, and it is not a good way to begin the professional relationship.

Setting Fees

When you set fees, a number of matters should be considered thoughtfully and proactively. These include prevailing fees charged by clinicians in your area, your level of experience and expertise, how many other clinicians in the local area provide comparable services, and the population you plan to serve, together with the likely ability of members of that population to pay for needed services. This is in keeping with Standard 1.13(a), Payment for Services, of the NASW (1999) Code of Ethics, which states: "When setting fees, social workers should ensure that the fees are fair, reasonable, and commensurate with the services provided. Consideration should be given to the clients' ability to pay."

As mentioned previously, fees should be set before one's first contact with a new client. It would be inappropriate to inform clients of the fees for services after the service is provided. Informing clients of the fees after seeing how they dress or what car they drive and basing the fee on your perception of their level of affluence would be patently unethical. Discussions of fees, payment options, and the like should be set in written office policies, they should be included in each client's informed-consent process, and this information should be shared with potential clients before the first session. Clinicians with websites often put their policies and forms online for clients to print and fill out before their first appointment. These suggestions are in keeping with the APA (2010a) Ethics Code's Standard 6.04(a), Fees and Financial Arrangements, which states: "As early as is feasible in a professional or scientific relationship, psychologists and recipients of psychological services reach an agreement specifying compensation and billing arrangements."

Because relationships with clients are built on trust, it is vital that the formation of this trusting relationship begin even before the first in-person contact. Furthermore, by sharing needed information with clients, to include fees, financial policies, and financial arrangements, we actively assist them to make informed decisions about participation in the professional relationship, helping to promote their autonomous functioning.

Anticipating a Client's Financial Limitations

In keeping with a focus on each client's best interests, the initial assessment of clients should not be limited solely to their clinical needs. Clients' financial situation should be openly discussed so that any financial limitations that might have an impact on their ability to participate in treatment may be addressed from the outset. Although all possible situations and circumstances can never be fully anticipated, having such a discussion with clients may also sensitize clients to these issues and highlight to them the need to be proactive should any change in their finances occur during the course of treatment.

Standard 6.04(d), Fees and Financial Arrangements, of the APA (2010a) Ethics Code makes this clear in stating: "If limitations to services can be anticipated because of limitations in financing, this is discussed with the recipient of services as early as is feasible." This discussion should address the nature of the anticipated financial difficulties, whether it is likely to be temporary or permanent, and whether there are other options to consider that might help make it easier for the client to afford treatment. Similarly, Standard A.10.b., Establishing Fees, of the ACA (2005) Code of Ethics includes the following statement:

> In establishing fees for professional counseling services, counselors consider the financial status of clients and locality. In the event that the established fee structure is inappropriate for the client, counselors assist clients in attempting to find comparable services of acceptable cost.

Financial limitations should be assessed in the initial session, and an appropriate treatment plan that takes these financial limitations into consideration should be developed (Knapp & VandeCreek, 2006). For example, developing a plan for 9 to 12 months of weekly psychotherapy sessions for an individual who can only afford 9 to 12 psychotherapy sessions would be inappropriate. When you perceive that the client's treatment needs exceed her or his financial resources, other options and treatment alternatives need to be discussed openly. The result of this discussion may be that the client is referred to another professional or program that is better able to work within his or her financial limitations, you could provide treatment to the client but with more limited treatment goals, or you might provide treatment to the client, making alternative financial arrangements so that he or she can afford to participate in treatment.

The pros and cons of each option should be openly discussed during the informed-consent process with each client. Furthermore, it is recommended that clinicians discuss fees and insurance participation during the first telephone contact with the prospective client. Insurance benefits may need to be verified ahead of time so that you know (or can estimate) what the client's financial liability will be.

Workers Compensation

Clients who experience an injury on the job may find that their treatment is not covered through their health insurance. Rather, it may be expected that the employer's workers compensation coverage will be responsible for any mental health care that is needed as a result of the injury. Each state has different workers compensation rules, and it is necessary for the clinician to be aware of these rules as they apply to the provision and reimbursement of services. Such services must be preauthorized, traditional confidentiality rules may not apply (e.g., in many states, treatment records are part of an "open system"), certain requirements must be met to be reimbursed (e.g., submission of treatment records with each invoice), fees may be set by a state agency or regulatory commission, clients may not be charged any co-pays or be billed for cancellations or no-shows, and care may only be authorized for curative treatment and not for palliative care. In addition, once it has been determined that the client has reached "maximum medical improvement," authorization (and payment) for services may cease immediately (with no sessions allowed for the termination process). Those working in this system must understand these policies so that each may be fully explained to the client. If care is to be continued past when it is authorized, discussions must take place regarding how the client will pay for this care.

The Role of Noninsurance Third Parties

During the informed-consent process, the role of any third parties should be made clear because they may have an impact on the treatment relationship. Third parties may include (a) parents or guardians who plan to pay for a client's treatment or whose insurance will be used to help cover the costs of the mental health services or (b) government agencies or legal authorities if treatment is mandated or required by law or the courts.

It is essential that the role and level of involvement in the mental health services to be provided is clarified from the outset and included in the informed-consent agreement. At times, the individual receiving the mental health service is not the one who accepts responsibility for payment for these services. However, as with all treatment agreements, it is best to have all parties sign a written agreement that specifies their roles and responsibilities, before the professional services being provided. It is recommended that verbal promises from the client about who will pay for treatment not be used. Statements such as "My step-dad said you should just bill him. He'll take care of everything" have no legal bearing and are not enforceable. When providing professional services to children of divorced parents, it may be important to review the settlement agreement to determine which parent is actually responsible for fees and to have a signed agreement with that parent.

There are times when treatment is for a diagnosis that ordinarily would be covered by an individual's insurance policy but the request for services came from a third party, such as the justice system. For example, although a client may have a diagnosis of intermittent explosive disorder, treatment may not be reimbursed if the counseling was court-ordered, such as the result of an arrest for a road-rage incident. Another example may be court-ordered alcohol abuse counseling following an arrest for driving while intoxicated. Insurance companies often do not consider these treatments "medically necessary" but to be forensically related. Clients have a right to be aware of reimbursement matters before initiating treatment.

When a third party requests or mandates mental health services for one's client, it is important that each party's responsibilities be fully discussed and documented from the outset. This should include responsibility for payment as well as access to treatment information. At times, a third party that accepts financial responsibility for an individual's treatment will assume that this brings with it certain rights or privileges, such as access to confidential treatment information or even the right to influence treatment planning and goal setting. As the ACA (2005)

Code of Ethics states in Standard B.3.d., Third Party Payers, "Counselors disclose information to third party payers only when clients have authorized such disclosure" (p. 8). Carefully addressing these matters in the informed-consent process and ensuring each party's understanding of agreed-on roles and responsibilities before the services are provided will help prevent misunderstandings and untoward effects as the professional relationship proceeds.

This informed-consent process becomes especially complicated when the identified patient is an adolescent. Barnett (2010) discussed ethical and legal aspects of working with this patient population and suggests that the way confidential information will be shared with parents be highlighted at the beginning of treatment. In certain jurisdictions, parents may have full access to their adolescent's treatment records, and in other jurisdictions no access at all. For example, in several states, adolescents aged over 14 years have the right to consent to their own treatment and thus to make treatment decisions to include regulating confidentiality; in other states, those aged 16 and older have this right. This can result in a situation in which an adolescent is admitted to a treatment program that is being paid for through the parent's insurance (with parents paying for the portion not covered by the insurance) but the professional staff is not allowed to share any information with the parents because the adolescent declines to provide this authorization. Although the therapeutic merits of such a system can be debated, the point is that it is important for treating professionals to provide informed consent about treatment and billing to all of the relevant parties so they understand their rights, obligations, and responsibilities from the outset.

Raising Fees

Like all others in business, mental health professionals have a range of expenses that may have an impact on their ability to remain viable and to earn a reasonable living. Expenses such as rent, utilities, telephone, insurance, and staff salaries are each likely to increase over time. Accordingly, mental health professionals will periodically need to increase the fees they charge. The possibility of such increases should be included in the informed-consent agreement so that clients will be able to factor these potential increased costs into their financial planning. For example, clinicians may include in the informed-consent agreement that all fees charged increase by 10% on January 1 of each year.

An alternative approach is to increase fees on an as-needed basis and to provide clients with advanced notice of doing so. Advanced notice is vital because some clients may not be able to afford increased fees. For these clients, the extra time may be used to consider other treatment options and to make alternative arrangements. We generally recommend 60 days notice, but this may be affected by factors that include the length of the client's treatment thus far and the client's financial situation. Furthermore, this should be fully discussed with the client and documented in his or her treatment record.

Mental health professionals certainly may increase their fees periodically, but they must remember to do so in a manner that is not exploitative of clients. Furthermore, in keeping with Standard 6.04(c), Fees and Financial Arrangements, of the APA (2010a) Ethics Code, "Psychologists do not misrepresent their fees." Accordingly, it would never be appropriate to charge one fee when a client enters treatment and then as soon as the treatment relationship is developed, dramatically increase the fee without notice.

When Clients Do Not Pay Agreed-On Fees

In addition to having a clear policy in place that addresses charges for missed appointments and charges for treatment sessions cancelled without adequate notice, it is also important to address the issue of unpaid bills with clients. The APA (2010a) Ethics Code states in Standard 6.04(e) that

> if the recipient of services does not pay for services as agreed, and if psychologists intend to use collection agencies or legal measures to collect the fees, psychologists first inform the person that such measures will be taken and provide that person an opportunity to make prompt payment.

Similar guidance is provided in the ACA (2005) Code of Ethics in Standard A.10.c., Nonpayment of Fees, which states,

> if counselors intend to use collection agencies or take legal measures to collect fees from clients who do not pay for services as agreed upon, they first inform clients of intended actions and offer clients the opportunity to make payment.

However, the prudent mental health professional will endeavor to use a preventive approach to addressing payment concerns rather than allow a client to build up a large outstanding balance owed. The first step is to address fees and payment requirements in the initial informed-consent discussion and include it in the written financial agreement. It is also recommended that a maximum allowable outstanding balance be specified in this agreement. For example, the clinician may inform clients that the maximum outstanding balance allowed is the equivalent of three sessions. Should the client's balance begin to grow, the clinician needs to remind the client of this agreement and discuss with him or her any difficulties that are present with regard to making payments. If, despite these reminders, that level of outstanding balance is reached, the clinician should openly discuss relevant concerns with the client and offer appropriate options. Such options include paying off the balance in full, working out a payment plan agreement, increasing the amount of time between treatment sessions, agreeing to a reduced fee either permanently or for an agreed-on period of time, referring the client to another professional or to a facility that offers a sliding fee scale or pro bono services, or some combination of these (e.g., allowing the client to pay a reduced fee, with the promise of the outstanding balance being paid at a specified rate over time after treatment is completed). Of course, the client's stated reasons for not paying agreed-on fees in a timely manner may affect the clinician's decision making on the best course of action. For example, one may respond quite differently to a client who recently lost her job and her health insurance than to a client who keeps forgetting his checkbook and makes continued promises to pay the fees owed but fails to do so.

Some clinicians may view these possible options with skepticism because of concerns about being accused of abandoning clients. It is important that mental health professionals understand that their obligation is to take actions to reasonably ensure that their clients' treatment needs are adequately addressed, not that they must personally provide ongoing treatment to a client indefinitely, even if the client is not paying for services as had been agreed-on in the informed-consent process.

As the ACA (2005) Code of Ethics states in Standard A.11.c., Appropriate Termination, "Counselors may terminate a counseling relationship when . . . clients do not pay fees as agreed upon." Further, Standard A.11.a., Abandonment Prohibited, states that "Counselors do not abandon or neglect clients in counseling. Counselors assist in making appropriate arrangements for the continuation of treatment . . . following termination."

Further guidance is found in the NASW (1999) Code of Ethics in Standard 1.16(c), Termination of Services, which states,

> Social workers in fee-for-service settings may terminate services to clients who are not paying an overdue balance if the financial contractual arrangements have been made clear to the client, if the client does not pose an imminent danger to self or others, and if the clinical and other consequences of the current nonpayment have been addressed and discussed with the client.

Additionally, Standard 1.16(d) states, "Social workers who anticipate the termination or interruption of services to clients should notify clients promptly and seek the transfer, referral, or continuation of services in relation to the clients' needs and preferences."

These standards support the ability of clinicians to make alternative arrangements when clients do not pay for treatment as had been agreed on, when done in keeping with ethical standards, and with attention to the client's ongoing treatment needs. However, it is clear that mental health professionals should never abruptly terminate clients' treatment when they are in crisis; clinical needs must be placed before financial gain. Addressing each client's ongoing clinical needs in a manner consistent with our obligation to "First, do no harm" (see Principle A: Beneficence and Nonmaleficence, APA, 2010a) can be done while ensuring that one does not have to provide clinical services indefinitely without being appropriately compensated (Younggren & Gottlieb, 2008).

When considering the option of using a collection agency or a small claims court, it is important for the mental health professional to remain cognizant of each client's particular circumstances. At times, clients may lose their ability to afford ongoing treatment. For example, clients may lose their jobs or health insurance benefits, or they may have unexpected expenses, such as those due to an illness or accident. Although all mental health professionals have the right to be fairly compensated for all services provided, they must at the same time be sensitive to their clients' financial circumstances.

Furthermore, mental health professionals should never terminate treatment solely for financial reasons. Clinical need must always be considered when making such decisions (Younggren & Gottlieb, 2008). Although no mental health professional is required to meet each client's every need, we are required to take reasonable steps to ensure that clients' treatment requirements are appropriately met and that clients are not abandoned (Vasquez, Bingham, & Barnett, 2008).

Should one wish to use a small claims court or collection agency to collect fees owed by a client, it is best to first discuss this with him or her and try to work out a mutually agreeable plan. If one decides to take this route, the client must first be informed of this possibility (in addition to the initial informed consent) and be offered options for making restitution in a reasonable and agreed-on time period. If this does not prove effective, the client is then informed of the action to be taken.

Although Standard 6.04(b), Fees and Financial Arrangements, of the APA (2010a) Ethics Code allows for the use of collection agencies and the use of small claims courts to collect fees owed by clients, risk management specialists have emphasized that the use of these means of collecting fees is often seen as antagonistic by clients and former clients (Bennett et al., 2006). These authors highlighted that clients who were previously pleased with the treatment received suddenly can find fault with it and file a malpractice suit or a complaint through a licensing board when they receive notice of a collections proceeding or of a legal action against them. In these cases, the amount of money spent defending oneself against these complaints typically far exceeds the amount one was trying to recover. Thus, prevention is deemed a much better approach for addressing fees owed by clients. However, should a collection agency be used, it is important to ensure that all requirements of one's ethics code are met, that the process be openly discussed with the client in advance of taking this action, that all such discussions be documented, that these discussions be followed up with written correspondence with copies kept in the treatment record, and that the collection agency is informed of acceptable and unacceptable practices. Furthermore, each client's confidentiality should be protected. The only information that should be shared with a collection agency is the client's name, the dates of service, and the fees owed.

Alternative Payment Methods

When clients are not able to pay for their needed treatment, mental health clinicians who still desire to provide the treatment have several options available to them. These include providing services on a pro bono basis, a sliding-scale basis, or through bartering.

PRO BONO SERVICES

Pro bono, or free, services are an option for all mental health professionals. Although this practice is not mandated in any of the mental health professions' ethics codes, it is encouraged when possible. The APA (2010a) Ethics Code Principle B: Fidelity and Responsibility includes the statement that "psychologists strive to contribute a portion of their professional time for little or no compensation or personal advantage." Similarly, in the introduction to Section A: The Counseling Relationship, the ACA (2005) Code of Ethics advises that "counselors are encouraged to contribute to society by devoting a portion of their professional activity to services for which there is little or no financial return (pro bono publico)" (p. 4). In its discussion of the value, Service, the NASW (2008) Ethics Code advises that "social workers are encouraged to volunteer some portion of their professional skills with no expectation of significant financial return (pro bono service)" (para. 20).

These suggestions are aspirational in nature. Mental health professionals must each decide if they can offer pro bono services, and if so, to how many clients and for what period of time, on the basis of their own unique financial circumstances. There is no ethical mandate to provide clients with services free of charge, but it is one option to consider for assisting clients experiencing significant financial hardship and who are in need of ongoing treatment. We also have a colleague who has found that doing an occasional pro bono forensic case has significantly enhanced his exposure and created significant goodwill in the courthouse, resulting in many additional referrals.

SLIDING FEE SCALE

A similar issue is that of a sliding fee scale: charging fees of varying amounts to clients on the basis of their ability to pay. Similar to pro bono services, this practice is never mandated but is an aspirational ideal that may be considered to enable clients to receive needed mental health services that they might not otherwise be able to afford. A sliding fee scale may be considered in situations in which clients who previously had paid the full fee for services are no longer able to afford this fee or whose insurance previously had provided coverage for treatment and no longer will do so. It also may be used as the initial payment method for clients in one's practice so that clients of limited means may be able to receive needed services.

When considering the use of a sliding fee scale, it is best to include the specific parameters of its use in a financial agreement that is included as part of the informed-consent process. Additionally, it is best if a consistent method for determining clients' fees is included in this agreement. For example, specific fees may be associated with certain reported household incomes. This practice may prove more effective than making individual determinations and decisions with every client who requests this fee option. The agreement should also specify any documentation of earnings or expenses that the clinician would want to review before making a fee determination. Finally, it is recommended that the issue of changes in the client's financial status be included in this financial agreement as well. Should the client no longer be in financial need and be able to afford a higher fee or even the full fee, that expectation should be clearly articulated in the agreement as well. Most clinicians will not be pleased to hear about a client's upcoming vacation to Disney World or see a client drive up in a new luxury car when providing services in good faith for a greatly reduced fee. It has been mentioned that the professional relationship is one that is built on trust, something that is relevant to both sides of the relationship.

BARTER

At times, the only way a client is able to afford needed mental health services is through the use of barter, payment in the form of goods or services by the client in exchange for the professional services. Although engaging in barter is not unethical per se, each of the mental health professions' ethics codes recommends caution when participating in it. These ethics codes do acknowledge that there are times when there may be no other way for clients to access needed treatment services, and there may be settings, such as some rural communities or with certain ethnic groups, where the use of barter is consistent with prevailing community standards.

As with other fee and payment arrangements, the use of barter should be discussed in detail in the informed-consent agreement. All barter arrangements should be discussed on an ongoing basis to ensure that neither party is feeling taken advantage of or exploited (Zur, 2007). Any difficulties experienced should be discussed openly as they arise. Furthermore, a specific written policy on barter is recommended to help ensure that it is applied consistently and to help prevent confusion or an adverse impact on the treatment relationship or process. It is also recommended that goods with an agreed-on value be chosen over the provision of services, for which disagreement over the quality and value could arise (Knapp & VandeCreek, 2008), and in situations in which an inappropriate multiple-relationship situation between the client and clinician may arise.

It is each mental health professional's ethical obligation to ensure that clients are not exploited by a barter arrangement. As the NASW (2008) Code of Ethics states, social workers may only engage in barter when it is "considered to be essential for the provision of services, negotiated without coercion, and entered into at the client's initiative and with the client's informed consent" (para. 75). Similarly, psychologists may only engage in barter with clients when "it is not clinically contraindicated" and "the resulting arrangement is not exploitative" (APA, 2010a, 6.05). The ACA (2005) Code of Ethics provides similar guidance and also adds that "counselors consider the cultural implications of bartering and discuss relevant concerns with clients and document such agreements in a clear written contract" (p. 6). The AAMFT (2001) Ethics Code calls for the establishment of a clear, written agreement and that there be an assurance that the professional relationship is not distorted as a result of the bartering arrangement.

Mental health professionals who engage in barter should also remember that they are receiving income (although it is not cash) for the services they are providing. As such, they are legally obligated to include the fair market value of the goods or services received in their income that is reported to the Internal Revenue Service and to pay taxes on what has been received. Failure to do so may bring with it significant tax and legal consequences.

Referrals and Fees

The process of making a referral of a client to another professional should always be motivated by the client's best interests. Referral decisions should be made based on the client's specific treatment needs and how well it appears that the new professional can meet those needs. A referral should not be motivated by the benefit of the referring professional. For example, the APA (2010a) Ethics Code in Standard 6.07, Referrals and Fees, states,

> When psychologists pay, receive payment from, or divide fees with another professional, other than in an employer–employee relationship, the payment to each is based on the services provided (clinical, consultative, administrative, or other) and is not based on the referral itself.

It is important that referrals not be motivated by possible financial gain for the referring practitioner but be based solely on the client's clinical and financial needs and interests. The payment or receipt of a fee for making or receiving a referral is considered a conflict of interest and not in keeping with the ethical standards of the mental health professions.

Conclusion

It is important that clinicians develop a working framework for billing and collecting of ethical practices that falls within legal guidelines. In developing procedures for this aspect of their business, we think it is important that clinicians attend to each of the following:

- Be familiar with the ethical principles and standard of their profession.
- Understand that informed consent applies not only to clinical issues but also to financial issues of paying for services.
- Be prepared to begin the financial portion of the informed-consent process as early as possible, even before treatment begins.
- Anticipate, if possible, financial limitations of the client's being able to pay for treatment.
- Be able to communicate adequately, both verbally and in writing, all financial aspects of treatment, including what role an insurance company may play in paying for all or part of services provided.
- Have a set policy that is communicated to clients regarding possible increases in fees.
- Have a set policy that is communicated to clients about what will occur if they do not pay for fees that are owed for services provided.
- Consider, within ethical guidelines, alternative payment methods such as accepting a sliding fee or bartering, when appropriate.
- Understand that when making referrals on behalf of clients, the overarching concern is the client's best interest and not any financial or professional gain for making the referral.

The Financial Agreement Between You and Your Client | 3

At the outset of treatment, the clinician and client must develop a written financial agreement that specifies the framework for providing ethically competent mental health care in the context of sound business practices. This agreement should inform the client about not only the clinical aspects of entering into an assessment or psychotherapy relationship but also the business aspects of the treatment relationship. It is important that clinicians understand the twofold nature and goals of the financial agreement. Although it creates a contractual arrangement and focuses on fees and other business matters, it is also a collaborative process that forms the basis of a trusting, open, and therapeutic relationship. In addition to being essential for good treatment, written agreements are an essential risk-management strategy.

There is something unique and special about the delivery of mental health services, and the ethics codes of the mental health professions require that such a document be in place. Although such documents do not exist in other forms of health care practice (how frequently do physicians or dentists in private practice have you sign such an agreement?), mental health professionals are held to a higher standard, and our contractual obligations hold us accountable to our clients both clinically and in our business. Thus, our written financial agreement lays the framework for effective and ethical billing.

In this chapter, we discuss the nature of financial agreements, sources of resistance to implementing the financial agreement from either client or clinician, and ways to overcome this resistance.

What Is a Contract?

In this book, we use the term *financial agreement* to refer to the contract between clinician and client. To better understand the financial agreement, consider the nature of contracts in general. We sign contracts all of the time. We do so to purchase homes and automobiles, to remodel our houses, to lease an office, to have cell phone coverage, and even to obtain a credit card. Contracts are an everyday part of life.

In *Business Law* (of the Barron's Business Review series), Emerson (2009) viewed contracts as essentially being a legally enforceable agreement between parties. According to Emerson, there are four elements to a valid contract: (a) capacity of the parties, (b) mutual agreement on the terms of the contract, (c) "consideration" (e.g., something that is provided in exchange for something else), and (d) legality of the subject matter. He added that the agreement represents "a meeting of the minds" (p. 103) after the terms of the contract are negotiated and agreed on.

In describing capacity of the parties, Emerson (2009) noted that one must be legally competent to enter into the agreement. As it relates to the delivery of mental health services, this means that minors in states where they are not allowed to consent to their own treatment cannot enter into a contract for services, nor can those impaired for mental health reasons. In each case, a guardian must enter into the contract on behalf of these individuals. Thus, someone who is actively psychotic may not be able to agree to a contract with a mental health clinician. Merely obtaining an individual's signature on a document will not result in a valid contract.

Emerson (2009) noted that there are two components of reaching mutual agreement in a contract: the offer and the acceptance. Two required components of the offer should be that it is sufficiently definite and that it is communicated to the other individual. As it relates to billing and collecting for mental health treatment, this means that in the financial agreement, the clinician should specify the length of sessions, general frequency of sessions, a no-show and cancellation policy, how billing will take place, the role (if any) of third party payors in the billing and collection process, a policy regarding unpaid balances due, and what is expected of the client in terms of his or her role in the billing and collection process. The client must then accept the terms of the offer that is presented or ask to negotiate parts he or she would like to change. After this meeting of the minds takes place, the client must accept the agreement. To reduce ambiguity, it is always best to have a written financial agreement rather than an oral one. Imagine telling a client that your psychotherapy hours are 50 minutes but it is their understanding that an hour is 60 minutes. If this is not specified from the beginning, the client may become angry when the clinician winds the session down before the client expects. A written agreement will also prove valuable should aspects of it need to be implemented and a client has a different recollection of the agreement than you do. For example, if a client who has been in counseling for several months and repeatedly cancels an appointment with little notice and is billed for them, it is helpful to have a written financial agreement to refer back to when reminding the client of your billing policy for missed or cancelled appointments.

Emerson (2009) stated that "consideration" is based on the concept of quid pro quo, or "something for something." In the case of the mental health practice, this is the clinician providing a service (e.g., psychotherapy, assessment, consultation) and receiving something in return from the client (e.g., payment) for doing so. The clinician communicates his or her fees for specific services and then the client agrees to pay this fee. In some instances, a third party may agree to pay all or part of the fee on behalf of the client, but the client is responsible to ensure that this fee is paid. It should be emphasized that even when insurance is involved, the financial agreement is between the client and the clinician, not between the insurer and the clinician. If the client is ultimately responsible for the fees charged (e.g., if the insurance only covers part of the fee, the client is responsible for the rest), this should be made clear in the written financial agreement as part of the informed-consent process.

Emerson (2009) stated that violations of law may nullify the enforceability of a contract. As it relates to mental health practice, this means that if clinicians are providing services that are not allowed under statutory law, the client may not have to keep up his or her end of the agreement (e.g., pay the fee). For example, consider the case of a licensed clinician supervising an unlicensed associate. The associate provides a clinical service under the clinician's supervision, but the clinician submits a request to an insurance company for the services provided, indicating or implying that the clinician provided the clinical services (not the associate). This would constitute fraudulent behavior. If this is discovered, it could be argued that whatever fees the client paid for the services should be returned and whatever fees were still due should be forgiven because of the violation of law invalidating the contract between the clinician and the client.

Emerson (2009) also explained that contracts entered into as a result of "undue influence" are not enforceable over the objection of the victim.

Emerson describes several types of confidential relationships (including doctor and patient) in which

> the person occupying a superior position, that is, one of trust, should be acting in the interest of the other person; hence any contract that is in reality for the former's benefit, and not for the latter's, is presumed to be tainted with undue influence and therefore voidable. (p. 111)

In the case of a mental health practice, this type of undue influence may take many forms. As an example, we live in a free-market system based on capitalism. As such, it could be argued that clinicians should be able to charge whatever they would like for their services. However, it might be considered undue influence if a private practitioner charges a client $1,000 per session when this is more than 3 times the going rate for even the most expensive clinicians in their area. Another example would be if a clinician purchases expensive biofeedback equipment and then decides that all of his or her clients are in need of 12 biofeedback sessions regardless of their diagnosis and level of psychological functioning. If the clinician "sells" the benefits of biofeedback to the clients, the purchaser is not in a position to determine whether such treatment is in his or her best interest. As can be seen, treatment decisions should be clinically motivated, not fiscally motivated—that is, they should be based on each client's actual treatment needs and best interests.

Appendix A provides a sample financial agreement between a clinician and a client. The strength of this document lies in its lack of ambiguity regarding billing and collecting. Specific fees are delineated for services provided, how these fees may be paid, what it means to be an in-network or out-of-network provider, how the clinician will bill insurance on behalf of the client, the role a managed care company may play in reimbursement, specific no-show or late-cancellation policies, other fees that may be due, and how unpaid debt will be handled.

Resistance to Implementing and/or Following the Written Financial Agreement

From a procedural point of view, billing and collecting should be an easy process. The clinician learns the procedures, explains them to the clients, applicable forms are submitted to insurance companies, and then the clinician receives payment. However, what seems so simple can actually become complicated because of either clinician or client resistance to making the process smooth and easy. Part of this problem is structural to our profession (e.g., there are few, if any, graduate courses in Private Practice 101), whereas others are personal or clinical. If this form of resistance can be identified, then corrections can be made in the billing and collecting process. To the extent that these resistances may compromise ethical decision making, overcoming them may also reduce ethical transgressions or the commissions of fraudulent behavior.

LACK OF TRAINING IN BUSINESS

How many of you reading this book received an A in your graduate course, Developing a Private Practice? Likely few of you answered that you indeed received such a fine grade. This is not because it is a difficult course but rather because few graduate training programs offer such a course in their curricula.

Because of a lack of training in graduate school, most mental health clinicians are not adequately prepared for their role as business people. Most clinicians likely learn on the fly about the business aspects of operating a practice—learning from other clinicians, attending workshops, or reading a book. Ethical and effective billing and collecting of fees for services is an essential component of making the small business of mental health practice profitable. Unfortunately, clinicians are rarely exposed to this important aspect of practice. In addition to enrolling in a graduate school course on the topic when this is available, clinicians are encouraged to attend workshops on billing and collecting, offered by both by the insurers and by clinicians who conduct "Business of Practice" seminars, so the rules and best practices may be learned directly. In addition, early-career clinicians should consider hiring a senior clinician as a consultant to ensure that all billing and collecting is done accurately, legally, and ethically. For psychologists, resources of the American Psychological Association Practice Organization and of Division 42 (Psychologists in Independent Practice) can be invaluable in learning more about this aspect of their businesses (see the Division 42 website: http://www.42online.org).

TRANSFERENCE

Clients bring their own issues and concerns regarding money in general, and paying for psychotherapy in particular, into the consulting room. Some clients want to pay nothing out of pocket for their treatment and have the expectation that their health insurance (or some other third party) will pay 100% of their costs, or that at most they will have a small co-pay. Other clients who prefer to maintain privacy may choose to pay 100% of the fee out of pocket so that no third party can have access to their confidential information. Despite signing a financial agreement as part of the informed-consent process at the beginning of treatment indicating that they will be charged and expected to pay for no-shows or late cancellations (e.g., not due to an emergency situation), some clients expect their psychotherapist to waive this fee because no service was delivered. Many clients have ambivalence about paying for psychotherapy because they may confuse this professional relationship with having a "good friend." Some clients cannot afford to pay the clinician's full fee and may be reluctant to ask for a reduction or to work out a payment plan. They may feel they are insulting the clinician if they ask for special accommodation. Some clients may expect the psychotherapist to work on a sliding-scale basis that fits their income, family size, and spending habits. After all, "they are rich doctors and can afford it." Some clients may run up considerable debt spending money on luxuries but be reluctant to place payment for psychotherapy on a credit card.

Each of these issues represents an intrapsychic variable that contributes to how clients think about fees and their responsibility to pay for psychotherapy or assessment services they are purchasing. These transference responses are grist for the mill of the psychotherapy that is taking place. Lanza (2001) noted that although "money is a taboo subject, it is also a royal road to unconscious material" (p. 71). Thinking psychodynamically, Herron (1995) stated that the fee is a definite avenue into the entire issue of clients' feelings about money that in turn is reflective of clients' attitudes about themselves and others. When the clinician has a specific fee policy, clients are consistently provided with opportunities to discuss the reactions to these fee policies (e.g., when they do not bring their co-pay for that day, begin to run up a balance due, will not follow-up if an insurance company fails to pay the clinician on time).

Herron (1995) elaborated on several advantages of having fees for psychotherapy. First, he stated that the collection of fees for direct service can be a motivator for clinicians to be diligent and do a good job. Second, because clinicians are being paid directly by someone who is purchasing a service, fees require clinicians to take responsibility for their work. Because a transaction is taking place, clients will expect a high level of care and professionalism. Third, Herron noted that fees are helpful in defining the professional nature of the relationship; thus, boundaries are placed on the relationship between the client and clinician. He viewed the clinician as a service provider who is having that service purchased by a consumer and that both operate under the rules of a professional relationship.

COUNTERTRANSFERENCE

Hayes (2004) defined countertransference as "therapist reactions to clients that are based on the therapist's unresolved conflicts" (p. 23). Gelso and Hayes (2001) suggested that countertransference that is not understood is likely to have a negative impact on the psychotherapy process. Further, countertransference that is managed well can help facilitate a positive treatment outcome. These authors identified five factors that are related to countertransference management: self-insight, self-integration, anxiety management, empathy, and conceptualizing ability.

In an earlier work (Walfish & Barnett, 2008), we stated the first principle of private practice success as follows: "You need to resolve the conflict between altruism and being a small business owner" (p. 8). If clinicians do not resolve this issue, they will be prone to financial mismanagement of their business and may place themselves at risk for ethical lapses, boundary transgressions, and possibly engaging in fraudulent behavior. As Gelso and Hayes (2001) suggested, these behaviors may be a result of poor countertransference management. Shapiro and Ginzberg (2006) stated that "difficulties managing financial arrangements are often attributed to therapists' conflicts over altruism and greed" (p. 479). Along these lines Herron (1995) opined,

> Therapists are prone to play artful dodger when it comes to fees. They need to get paid, and they want to get paid, but they do not want patients to be aware of therapists' desires for money. Unfortunately there is a high degree of sharing the misconception that money must tarnish the psychotherapeutic relationship. (p. 12)

Herron further stated, "A major problem in giving fees their appropriate emphasis is still the reaction that the emphasizer is crass and uncaring" (p. 15).

We heard Bill Cosby once comment, "The reason that grandchildren and grandparents get along so well is because they have a common enemy." We think that clients and psychotherapists often have a similar relationship with insurance companies. That is, at times, they may mutually plan and plot to have the insurer pay for services when they are not part of the contract that either the client or the clinician has with the insurance company. Gresham (2009) provided the example that many insurance companies will not pay for V-code diagnoses such as Marital and Partner Problem or Parent–Child Relational Problem. Therefore, when a client will not want to, or cannot, pay for these services out of pocket, the clinician may bill with a Current Procedural Terminology code that is reimbursable (e.g., individual psychotherapy vs. marital psychotherapy) or a diagnosis that is reimbursable (e.g., Adjustment Disorder with Depressed Mood vs. a V-code). Gresham stated that although such actions likely are intended to be helpful to the client, when they occur, the clinician and client collude against the third party corporate entity. Although few people will cry over an insurance company making less money, this type of behavior is unethical and illegal. In addition, this is also poor modeling by the clinician for their client of how to problem solve a difficult situation.

Gresham's (2009) observation is borne out by research indicating that a client's diagnosis may vary depending on whether he or she is paying privately or having a managed care company pay the professional fee

(Kielbasa, Pomerantz, Krohn, & Sullivan, 2004; Pomerantz & Segrist, 2006). In this same vein, Sharfstein, Towery, and Milowe (1980) found that diagnoses submitted to insurance companies are often inaccurate because of concerns about patient confidentiality and concerns about the potential consequences of having such a diagnosis on one's record. Further, these authors stated that "because of the social stigma and often pejorative connotations attached to certain psychiatric diagnoses many clinicians are concerned that writing down a diagnosis which the patient may see can have adverse effects on the therapeutic process" (p. 72).

On a recent listserv discussion, several clinicians noted that they were reluctant to diagnose a client with an Axis II personality disorder for fear that the client would be upset with such a diagnosis and leave treatment. Once again, the ethical mandate is to provide accurate diagnoses when submitting claims to insurance companies. It is also possible that clients will be unhappy with these (accurate) diagnoses, become upset with the clinician, and leave treatment. Because clients provide income for the clinician this may be a situation that the clinician, consciously or unconsciously, wants to avoid. As part of a true informed-consent process, clinicians should discuss the diagnosis with the client and the ramifications of such a diagnosis being placed on an insurance document. Unfortunately, the diagnosis is what the diagnosis is, and the procedure code is what the procedure code is; it cannot be altered either to have a third party pay a bill that is actually a client's responsibility or to keep a clinician from having unfilled openings in his or her schedule.

Utilizing Gelso and Hayes's (2001) five factors of countertransference management as they apply to fees and the collection of fees may be helpful in reducing the likelihood of ethical transgressions. In terms of the first factor, *self-insight*, it is important that clinicians understand their own relationship with money and their role as a professional in charging (not inexpensive) fees for helping others. Rodino (2005) suggested that self-examination of these matters can be helped by exploring family history, role models, fear of success, a feeling of being unworthy of financial success, and possible conflicts with religious, ethical, and moral upbringing. Grodzki (2004) urged social workers to "make peace with money" and, along with Rodino, saw the need to resolve childhood concerns that may influence the development of a successful business.

According to Gelso and Hayes (2001), the second factor, *self-integration*, refers to the clinician having an intact character structure, and this allows the clinician to have good ego boundaries. This will prevent overidentification with clients in their battle with the insurance company and an ability to avoid collusion by changing diagnoses or procedure codes.

Gelso and Hayes's (2001) third factor is *anxiety management*. Gresham (2009) has found that many clinicians who are avoidant in their personal money management will have a more difficult time initiating discussions and dealing with clients in relation to fees and money in their practice. Getting comfortable initiating money conversations with clients is the first step in building skills in this area. Herron (1995) suggested that clinicians may be so uncomfortable with clients' reactions about fees that they may try and keep them as invisible as possible. We are aware of many clinicians who are so uncomfortable with discussing financial matters with their clients that they delegate this to their office staff or an outside billing service.

Fees are part of psychotherapy in private practice, and clinicians must become as comfortable discussing this issue as any other personal material that may be relevant to treatment. Sommers (2000) presented an interesting discussion regarding the "enforcement" of no-show policies in which clients have agreed to pay for sessions that they miss for nonemergent reasons. She noted, "Therapists think of themselves as helpers, not enforcers, so strong feelings can arise when it becomes necessary to stand firm on policy requiring payments for missed sessions" (p. 56). In this article, Sommers self-disclosed her own journey in becoming comfortable with keeping to the promise or assurance of the policy that was agreed on at the beginning of treatment.

It is also important to note that firmly and consistently enforcing boundaries in the treatment relationship and treatment process is clinically important. Failure to follow through with stipulations of the written financial agreement may be clinically relevant and significant for clinician and client alike. It may not be in a client's best interest clinically for a clinician to avoid discussing finances and not to follow through with collecting fees. This practice could actually reinforce maladaptive patterns from the client's life and be countertherapeutic. Additionally, enforcing treatment agreements and maintaining appropriate boundaries may be a way for clinicians to model appropriate and adaptive behavior for clients. Put another way, it would seem that most clinicians would not want to model avoidance behaviors in the face of discomfort to their clients.

Gelso and Hayes's (2001) fourth factor is *empathy*. Sitkowski and Herron (1991) found that compared with clients, clinicians have differing attitudes about money. Clinicians place an emphasis on its potential for providing security, including protection from anxiety generated by money. Herron (1995) noted that appropriate sensitivities to the client's feelings about financial matters is essential, especially given how finances can be an emotionally charged issue for the client. He suggested an interpersonal style that is low key yet firm and consistent.

Gelso and Hayes's (2001) fifth and final factor is *conceptualizing ability*. It is important for the clinician to understand what role the fee plays in psychotherapy and what transference responses related to fee payment or nonpayment may arise during the course of treatment.

Paying attention to a countertransference response is important, whether it be sexual attraction to a client, anger or disappointment in a client, or the financial aspect of the treatment relationship. Mental health practitioners need to resolve any underlying conflicts they may have with regard to money and success. Feelings of guilt over success and benefitting financially from the suffering of others must be worked through and resolved for someone to be an effective and helpful clinician. Thus, understanding the meaning and role of money in one's family of origin and resolving any related conflicts that may be present are essential for ethical and effective functioning in the psychotherapy relationship. If clinicians have difficulty managing the billing and collections aspect of their practice, we suggest they seek out supervision or consultation from a trusted colleague; if the issue is more deep-seated, they should explore this in the context of personal psychotherapy.

Gender Issues

We believe that because of socialization and cultural training, female clinicians often have more difficulty than male clinicians with the financial aspects of private practice. Lasky (1984) found male clinicians to focus more on the practical aspects of amount of income generated and financial support of their families than on any internal conflict over money that might be present. However, she found female psychotherapists to have an "acute awareness of the conflict and to be deeply pained by it" (p. 294). Two of these conflicts centered around (a) needing the financial income for themselves and their families versus appearing greedy and (b) the tendency to focus more on the client's financial needs than on their own. One survey focused on differences in fee setting by male and female psychologists in a Colorado county (Newlin, Adolph, & Kreber, 2004) and found no differences between the sexes, but the authors cautioned that the results might not generalize on a national level because the sample size was small and localized to one county.

In the excellent book *Women Don't Ask*, Babcock and Lashever (2003) examined sex differences in feelings about money and work. If discussing money and negotiation is an issue, we suggest consulting this fascinating read to learn more about the deleterious effects of avoiding this problem in terms of self-worth and actual money lost (or not earned). It is essential that mental health practitioners resolve the conflict between helping others in the context of a caring and meaningful relationship and being in a business in which one goal is financial success.

Clinicians should question their own judgments and biases. For example, when you hear of a clinician who owns a large multisite practice that employs more than 30 clinicians, do you think of a good clinician who is caring and compassionate and who is helping to ensure that those in need are able to receive needed services? Or are you picturing a businessperson who is focused on making money and who puts profits and greed over others' needs? Self-reflection, self-awareness, and honesty with oneself about these matters and working through them early in one's career are strongly recommended. We do not see business success as inconsistent with clinical expertise and compassion. In fact, being financially successful can assist the clinician in being able to offer services to some clients who might not otherwise be able to afford them.

Conclusion

The financial agreement serves as a contract between clinician and client and functions as the basis for how these services are compensated. In addition to a financial agreement, there are also ethical considerations unique to the provision of mental health services that need to be taken into consideration through a comprehensive informed-consent process. The financial agreement in particular, and the informed-consent process in general, help to ensure the ethical and effective provision of clinical services and to promote accountability; they also serve as effective risk-management strategies. Thus, we think it essential to do the following:

- address fees and financial arrangements in a written financial agreement that is a component of a comprehensive informed-consent process;
- understand the nature of contracts as they apply to a mental health practice;
- take the time to become knowledgeable in the business of practice, despite this not being part of graduate training;
- understand that clients not only have transference reactions to clinical issues but may also have transference reactions to paying for mental health services provided to them;
- understand that clinicians not only have transference reactions to clinical issues but may also have transference reactions to clients paying, or not paying, for mental health services that they have provided; and
- avoid colluding with a client against their insurance company.

The Nuts and Bolts of Getting Paid for Your Services

4

F ew clinicians who have a psychotherapy or assessment practice actually collect 100% of the fees that they charge. There is almost always going to be some amount of loss. This loss could be due to client irresponsibility, human error on the part of clinicians or their staff, or a humanitarian decision to waive some fees that are due as a result of client hardship.

We have often thought that clients who do not meet their obligations spelled out in the financial agreement are in essence stealing from us. After all, we have in good faith delivered a professional service with the expectation of receiving an agreed-upon fee. However, we are also aware that not everyone is financially responsible with their other bills as well. Clients may not pay their credit card bill or fees due to other service providers such as physicians, accountants, or their utility company. Large businesses factor this loss into their overall business model as they plan for profits. For example, Visa knows that a certain portion of consumers will default on balances due. In deciding what interest rates to charge, this loss is taken into consideration. Nordstrom and Target estimate nonpayment of credit cards and losses from theft in their financial projections. The same concept applies to private practices, and we believe mental health clinicians should set up procedures to maximize collections and minimize loss.

Clinicians may be paid in one of two ways: directly by the client or by a third party, such as an insurance company. The simplest way for the clinician is to be paid directly by the client in what is commonly referred to as a *fee-for-service practice*. However, because most psychotherapy clients prefer to use their insurance benefits to help pay for all or a significant portion of their fee, the more common way that clinicians get paid is by billing the client's insurance company and then waiting for payment from it. Insurance companies usually pay most of the fee, and the clinician collects a co-pay from the client as well as any unpaid portion of their deductible that may be due.

The clinician must establish a set of procedures to be reimbursed for services provided. These procedures can be simple in a fee-for-service practice and complicated in a practice in which clinicians are providers for insurance companies. The purpose of this chapter is to expose clinicians to practical steps for optimizing billing and collecting of fees. We discuss billing in which insurance is not involved; billing in which insurance is involved (including the preauthorization process, verification of benefits, completing claim forms, and evaluating payments from insurance companies); collecting co-pays from clients, accepting credit card payments, and dealing with audits by insurance companies; and billing in special circumstances, such as Medicare and workers compensation.

Billing and Collecting in a Fee-for-Service Practice

A fee-for-service practice may be conceptualized as a "pay as you go" type of business transaction. After the fee is agreed on (as early as possible in the professional relationship), billing and collecting for services provided is a straightforward process.

Some clinicians collect their fee at the beginning of each session. Some collect the fee after the service is provided. These differences may be based on psychotherapeutic orientation or simply a preference for one over the other. Hunt (2006) suggested that by collecting fees at the beginning of the session, (a) problems related to failing to bring payment can be dealt with during the session and (b) the full focus of the session may be placed on clinical concerns rather than dealing with payment at the end of the clinical hour.

Fees may be collected by office support personnel or directly by the clinician. This, too, may be based on treatment orientation because some practitioners like to separate clinical issues from financial issues.

Some long-term psychotherapy clients may prefer to be billed monthly rather than to have to write a check for each appointment. We suggest this decision be made on a case-by-case basis, but clinicians must understand that if they are not paid each week, they are running the risk of not being paid for their services. This risk may be worth taking to increase customer satisfaction, especially if this is the client's preferred payment method. If the client has a credit card guaranty on file (discussed later in this chapter), then the clinician can be more confident that fees will be paid on a timely basis and that the client will not ever have a large unpaid balance due.

Careful record keeping is essential, and each clinician should keep a written record of all dates of service, fees charged, fees collected, and any amounts due. One should never trust one's memory of which clients forgot their checkbook and need to mail a check or pay next time. It is easy to lose track and mismanage fees owed if careful records are not kept. As mentioned in Chapter 3, it is also important to include in the financial agreement the maximum allowable outstanding balance for treatment to continue. Doing so, and following through with this policy, can help increase collections and minimize the risk of clients not paying sizeable outstanding balances.

There are two types of fee-for-service payments. One occurs when clients pay their bills and have no desire to be reimbursed by their insurance company. Some individuals do not want a paper trail indicating that they have ever sought mental health services. In the second instance, if clients have out-of-network benefits in their insurance policy, they may wish to be reimbursed by their insurance company for some (likely) or all (very unlikely) of what they paid for their psychotherapy or assessment sessions. In these cases, the clinician must provide the client with a superbill, which includes the name of the client, the diagnosis, the date of service, the service provided, and the amount charged for each service. The name of the clinician must also be included, and in some instances insurers require either a tax ID number for the clinician or a National Provider Identifier (NPI) number. A sample superbill may be found in Appendix B and can be easily designed with a word processing program.

In some instances, managed care companies will want the clinician to complete forms so that the client may be reimbursed. In such cases, we consider it a courtesy to clients to complete the forms so they can be reimbursed. One could rightfully charge for the time it takes to complete the forms, but the client may perceive this as being "nickel and dimed" by the clinician. As an alternative, we suggest taking a few minutes of session time to complete the forms so the client can then submit them.

Billing and Collecting When an Insurance Company Is Involved

When clients use insurance to pay for part or all of their psychotherapy, the process is more complex than for a fee-for-service practice. Although none of the steps are difficult, they do require attention to detail. In our previous book, *Financial Success in Mental Health Practice* (Walfish & Barnett, 2008), our Private Practice Principle Number 15 states: "While Not to the Point of Having a Disorder, It Is Helpful to Have Some Obsessive–Compulsive Tendencies When Dealing With Insurance Companies and Collecting Payments from Clients" (p. 126).

As noted earlier, one reason clinicians do not collect 100% of their fees is human error. Paying attention to the details of billing and collecting will optimize the amount of money earned by clinicians. We believe insurance and managed care companies rely on clinicians not turning billing in on time and not requesting preauthorization for services or reauthorization for additional services. Recently, Steve Walfish completed an evaluation with a client on a Saturday. On Monday morning, he called for authorization. The managed care company replied, "We will not pay you for these services because you did not request them ahead of time." By contractual arrangement with the insurance company, he could not bill the client either. These errors and oversights add to insurance company profits. By attending to the following concerns, you can avoid common problems with billing and collecting from an insurance company.

OBTAINING PREAUTHORIZATION AND VERIFYING BENEFITS

It is important that clinicians be aware of the contracts they sign with insurance companies to be a preferred provider or with managed care companies (MCCs). For some policies, called *open access*, no preauthorization for services is required. For others, the client must call the company ahead of time to have services authorized, and in some instances, the clinician must place this call. Some insurers and MCCs allow this to be completed online.

If clinicians call for preauthorization, they must first obtain identifying information from the client; otherwise the insurance company or MCC will not speak with them. This information includes (a) the name of the client, (b) the name of the insured, (c) the relationship to the insured (if not the client), (d) the date of birth of the client, (e) the home telephone number and address of the client, (f) the member or subscriber identification number, and (g) the name of the employer.

It is important to know exactly what is being authorized—that is, whether it is just an initial consultation (Current Procedural Terminology [CPT] Code 90801) or whether it is this consultation plus a certain number of psychotherapy sessions (CPT Code 90806). If the session numbers are limited in this authorization, it is important to know how to request further sessions if necessary and when (e.g., after the authorized sessions have been exhausted or two sessions prior?). It is important to understand that if the sessions are not authorized, the insurance company will not pay you for services provided and the cost will not be passed on to the client.

Most insurers and MCCs require preauthorization for psychological testing. Some may authorize a minimal number of hours (e.g., 3 or 4) without requesting any documentation; others require the completion of a form titled "Request for Psychological Testing" or something similar. Some allow this form to be completed online, whereas others require that the form be faxed to them. This form usually requires the clinician to state the current symptoms of the client, the purpose of the testing, why testing may be needed and what information may be gained from it as opposed to the information gathered in a clinical interview, the names of the tests to be completed, and the amount of time requested. A psychologist reviews this form and decides within company guidelines whether the testing will be authorized and, if so, how many hours will be authorized for reimbursement. If authorization is denied, this decision may be appealed to another level within the company. Contractually, however, the final decision lies with the insurer or MCC. In some instances, if services are denied, the psychologist may bill the client directly. This varies from contract to contract. Once again, it is important to be familiar with the details of the contract you have signed with the insurance company. If the client is to be billed directly for services declined by the MCC or insurer, then it is important to have the client acknowledge in writing that they want the clinician to perform the service even though their insurer has denied payment and that they will be financially responsible for the total cost of the services.

As part of the preauthorization process, it is important to understand the benefits of the client's policy. It is ethically important to know this information from the beginning of treatment. If clients are counting on insurance to help pay for treatment and the benefits have limitations that will preclude payment for the amount of treatment they likely need or if the co-pay or deductible is so high that it becomes a financial hardship, this must be planned for at the onset. For example, if the client has a high deductible (e.g., $1,000 per year) or a high co-pay (e.g., $50 per session) and they have no way to pay these monies, then alternative plans for treatment must be made. Discovering this in the middle of treatment could jeopardize the therapeutic alliance and can easily become problematic for the success of the treatment being provided. The client expects to receive services, and the clinician expects to be paid for those services. Both are reasonable positions to have but may not fit the reality of the situation.

When verifying benefits, it is important to obtain the following information:

1. Whether the plan has mental health benefits. Most group policies have such benefits, but many individual policies do not.
2. What the client's deductible is under the policy and whether there is a separate deductible for mental health services.
3. What portion of the deductible has been met.
4. What, if any, co-pay is due from the client for each session. If the co-pay is expressed in a percentage of allowed charges (as opposed to a specific dollar amount), then it is important to know the rate for which you contracted services with this insurance company or MCC. In rare instances, beyond a co-pay there is also an additional coinsurance portion that is due from the client. It appears that the difference between the two is solely semantic, and this enables the clinician to collect two fees from the client.
5. Whether there is a maximum number of sessions allowed per calendar year or whether there is an annual or a lifetime maximum dollar amount of benefits that may be paid on behalf of the client. Health insurance reform and the passage of parity legislation should eliminate these impediments, but the practical implementation of these policies has yet to be fully determined.

When verifying benefits, the person on the phone or the online correspondence that you receive will contain a disclaimer about possible noncoverage of benefits. Although you are "verifying benefits," the insurer or MCC is not "guaranteeing benefits" in this transaction. They may tell you that a person is covered, but the final determination is made when an insurance claim is submitted and reviewed. Insurers do not update their subscriber rolls on a daily basis. There will be cases in which a person may not be covered (e.g., left the job, did not pay a premium), and this change has not yet been made in the insurer's database. We have also had cases in which payment was made in error only to be discovered 6 to 12 months after the fact. If an error is made, the insurance company may ask for a refund of the payment. In some cases, there may be laws in one's jurisdiction that limit the insurer's ability to collect fees already paid if requested after a certain period of time. If such a request is received from an insurer, we recommend checking to see whether such a limit exists in your jurisdiction.

COMPLETING CLAIM FORMS

This aspect of the billing process is made easier if a computerized billing program is used. Each form has identifying information about the clinician and his or her practice that is entered only once and then kept in memory for all future claim submissions. Without such a system, the clinician must generate this same information on a repetitive basis for each claim submitted.

Appendix C provides a sample insurance claim form (CMS-1500). This form has four basic sections: (a) identifying information about the client, (b) authorization to provide information and to be paid directly, (c) a description of the services provided, and (d) identifying information about the clinician.

The basic information regarding the client that is needed includes (a) client name, date of birth, and address; (b) name of the subscriber (if different from the client) and relationship to the client; (c) an indication as to whether the care is a result of a work-related injury or motor vehicle accident (if this is the case, another type of insurance, e.g., workers compensation or automobile insurance policy, may be responsible for payment); and (d) the member or subscriber identification number, the group number of the employer, and the name of the employer. This last set of information may be found on the client's insurance card.

The authorization section covers two areas. First, the client must agree to authorize the release of medical or other information requested by the insurance company or other third party payors to facilitate claims processing. It is important that clients understand that insurance companies and MCCs reserve the right to ask for treatment records when they are to pay for part or all of the costs of an insured's mental health services. Although we have found the request for such records to be rare, it is best to review this possibility with clients as part of the informed-consent process. There are some clients who do not want a paper trail of such records and may opt to pay for psychotherapy out of pocket or not to enter psychotherapy when they learn of this potential threat to their privacy. Although they may not receive needed care (or at a minimum, payment of it by their insurer), it is their individual right to make this choice. Second, the client must authorize payment directly to the clinician. If this box is not signed, then the payment will go directly to the client. Note that if the clinician is a provider for an insurance company or MCC, most contracts preclude the clinician from collecting full payment from the client at the time of service, except for allowable deductibles and co-pays. That is, the clinician must wait the 2 to 6 weeks (usually 30 days) to be reimbursed by the insurance company or MCC for everything beyond the client's co-pay (after their annual deductible has been met).

The third section focuses on why the services were provided, where the services were provided, what services were provided, and the amount charged for services. This section includes a space for the name of the referring physician (if any) and the diagnosis of the client. This is followed by date of service and specific numeric codes for place and type of service. Computer billing programs have these listed in their databases. The most common place of service in private practice is an outpatient office (coded as 11), and there are codes for inpatient hospital, skilled nursing facility, inpatient psychiatric facility, and numerous others. A list of commonly used place of service codes may be found online (http://www.delphipbs.com/help/html/placesetup.htm). Next is the numeric CPT code, which describes the type of service. The most common mental health CPT codes are Initial Evaluation (90801), Psychotherapy 45–50 minutes (90806), Family Therapy With Patient Present (90847), Group Psychotherapy (90853), and Psychological Testing With Report (96101). A list of the most commonly used codes in private practice may be found online (http://www.thriveboston.com/counseling/mental-health-cpt-codes-for-professional-reference), and computer billing programs have these listed in their databases as well. The amount charged for services is also listed in this section. The amount placed in this column should be the usual and customary charges of the clinician and not the contracted discounted amount. When processing the claim, the insurance company will make the necessary adjustments in determining how much to pay the clinician on the basis of what was agreed to in the insurance company's contract with the clinician.

The fourth section focuses on the practitioner's personal information. It is simply a listing of your tax ID number, whether you accept assignment of benefits for claims, your address, and your NPI number. In addition, if the services were delivered outside of your office, there is a box to insert the name of the facility where they were provided.

A more detailed step-by-step guide for completing the form is presented in our previous book (Walfish & Barnett, 2008). For those psychologists who are members of the American Psychological Association and pay the Practice Assessment fee, a video showing how to complete this form is available on the Practice Directorate section of the American Psychological Association's website (http://www.apa.org).

SUBMITTING THE FORM

Claims forms may be submitted manually via the mail, electronically through a computerized billing system, or in some cases on the websites of the insurance company or MCC. These last two have an advantage over the former in that claims are generally paid faster and mistakes in billing can immediately be identified.

EVALUATING PAYMENTS RECEIVED

When the claim is paid, the check will be accompanied by an Explanation of Benefits (EOB). The EOB will list the date of service, type of service provided, amount billed by the clinician, the amount disallowed by the contract, the amount paid by the insurer, and the amount due from the client (co-pay). This document must be carefully scrutinized. Insurance companies make mistakes, and it is up to the clinician to follow up with them when they do to have mistakes corrected. It is most efficient to do this in writing rather than on the telephone and run the risk of being placed on hold for 10 minutes (and not have a written record of your efforts as well).

Claims may be denied for reasons such as the insurer not having authorization on file (even though you may have received authorization in writing), the insurer not being able find the subscriber in their system (even though you are looking at a copy of their insurance card), it appearing that the subscriber has other insurance coverage and the insurer has asked the client for information about this before paying on the claim (in which case you have to follow up with the client to make sure they contact the insurer), or for myriad other reasons. Each denial should be followed up with an explanation in writing to the insurance company about why the company should be paying the claim. Failure to follow up will result in the insurance company keeping the money.

BILLING SECONDARY INSURANCE

Some clients will have two insurance policies in effect. This may be due to a person working but also having had a previous career (e.g., military, government) and retaining the insurance as a lifetime benefit or a spouse or domestic partner having coverage through their employer and the client being included in their family plan. It is important for the clinician to determine which insurance policy is primary (usually the insurance associated with the current work position) and which is secondary. The primary insurance must first be billed with an CMS-1500 form. When the EOB is received from the primary insurance, the secondary insurance may then be billed. This insurance company will want to know what benefits were paid by the primary insurance company, so it is important to include a photocopy of this EOB when submitting the second claim.

COLLECTING THE CLIENT PORTION DUE

Rarely do insurance companies pay 100% of the fee due for providing services. There is usually a co-pay or coinsurance due to the clinician from the client. This may take the form of a specific dollar amount (e.g.,

$10, $15, $25) or a percentage of the allowed billable amount (e.g., 10%, 20%). These amounts vary from insurance company to insurance company and even within insurers from contract to contract. That is, for example, all Aetna policies are not the same, and co-pays due may differ for those Aetna subscribers working for Company X and those Aetna subscribers working for Company Y.

Most insurance cards will indicate whether there is a co-pay due and will express it in terms of a dollar amount or a percentage. If it is a percentage, this is computed on the basis of the discounted contracted fee that the clinician has agreed to with the insurance company and not the usual and customary fee charged. For example, if the clinician usually charges $100 per session but the contracted allowed amount by the insurance company is $ 70 and a 10% co-pay is due, then the client is responsible for only $7 per session (and the insurer should forward payment of $63 to the clinician).

It is best that co-pays be collected at the time the session takes place. This allows the clinician to maintain a positive cash flow (those $15 co-pays do add up by the end of the month), prevents a balance due from building up, and eliminates the need to send out follow-up bills for balances due. When the EOB is inspected, it may be found that the deductible had not been met or the co-pay was greater than expected. When this occurs, the client must be sent a follow-up bill. Computer billing programs can generate such an invoice. Our previous book (Walfish & Barnett, 2008) presented a simple word-processing format that may be used to generate an invoice. On the clinician's letterhead, a form may be developed that includes the client's name and address, type of service delivered (e.g.. psychotherapy), date of service, total amount charged, insurance discount, insurance payment received, direct payment received, and total balance due.

It is also recommended that a specific payment due date be included. If the client does not pay by that date, then a follow-up reminder should be sent out shortly thereafter. It is important to attempt to collect these monies for two reasons. First, the monies are due for services that have been rendered. It is a fee that the clinician is entitled to receive; routinely letting these amounts go uncollected will have a negative impact on the clinician's income. Second, as discussed later, it may give the appearance that the clinician is waiving co-pays or deductibles, which could be considered a fraudulent billing practice. A reasonable attempt must be made to collect these monies. Sending out three invoices would be considered reasonable, and if still unpaid, this should be documented in the client's chart.

An in-network provider may not "balance bill" a client for the difference between their usual and customary fee and what the contracted rate allows. For example, if a clinician's usual and customary fee is $100 per session, the contracted rate with the insurer is $80 and there is a $10 co-pay due, then the insurance company will send the clinician a check for $70. The clinician is only allowed to collect the $10 co-pay for a total payment of $80 for the session as specified in the contract with the insurance company. The $20 difference between the usual and customary fee ($100) and contracted fee ($80) may not be collected. This is not the case for out-of-network providers because no contracted rate has been agreed to with the insurer, and the entire fee may be collected (as per the clinician's financial agreement with the client). In the example cited earlier, if clients use out-of-network benefits, they should expect to receive a $70 check directly from the insurance company. However, their agreed-on fee with the clinician was $100, and therefore they would be paying $30 out of pocket for this session.

Clinicians cannot routinely waive co-pays for clients. To do so would be considered fraudulent by the insurance company. Government regulations regarding Medicare make it clear that routine waiver of deductibles and co-pays is illegal because "it results in (1) false claims, (2) violations of the anti-kickback statute, and (3) excessive utilization of items and services paid for by Medicare" (U.S. Department of Health and Human Services, 1994). Fernandez (1999) indicated that insurers consider waiving co-pays fraud because they are paying for 100% of the client's care rather than the actual portion (e.g., 80%) they have contracted to pay. Fernandez suggested that when the co-pay is waived, there is an incentive for clients to overuse services when the care is essentially free for them. He also indicated that insurers have found that health care providers who routinely waive co-pays are often guilty of inflating their fees and charging for services that were not rendered. This does not mean that you can never waive a co-pay for genuine financial hardship. Medicare regulations (U.S. Department of Health and Human Services, 1994) indicate that these fees can be waived on an occasional basis but not routinely. If a fee is being waived for financial hardship, it is important to document in the client's chart why this is being done.

Accepting Credit Cards

We strongly suggest that that clinicians consider accepting credit cards for payment of services. Psychologist Jessica Dolgan (2010) pointed to the "power of plastic" in operating a financially successful private practice. As a consultant to psychotherapy practices and owner of a billing and collection service for mental health clinicians, she has found significant increases in collections in a short period of time simply by adding this payment method. She indicated that clients will likely attend more sessions if credit card payment is a possibility (e.g., weekly instead of every 2 to 4 weeks); that it is easier to be paid for services provided, including co-pays and no-shows or late cancellations, if the client has agreed to place such charges on a credit card that the clinician gathers at intake; that some clients prefer paying all of their bills via credit card because of additional benefits to them (e.g., airline miles, cash back); and that when credit cards are used, it is easy to collect for past balances due. Thus, revenues increase, and the clinician and client are not faced with the dilemma of running up a large balance while still in the need of clinical services. There are fees charged to the clinician by the credit card company, but the greater benefit derived from using them may offset these charges.

A sample credit card guaranty form is provided in Appendix D. Essentially, this document allows the clinician to bill any unpaid charges to a client's credit card that is kept on file. For in-network clients, Steve Walfish bills the insurance company, receives payment back from the company, and then sends an invoice to the client for any balance due. A note is included indicating that if this balance is not paid within 14 days, the amount will be charged to the credit card on file "as per our agreement." Since implementing such a strategy, the amount of Steve's accounts receivable has been drastically reduced. It should be pointed out that this is not a fool-proof strategy. At times, Steve has found the credit card to be maxed out or rejected for some other reason. Some clients may not have or use credit cards either as a lifestyle decision or as a consequence of declaring bankruptcy. In such cases, Steve tells the client that he will have "to trust them" to pay their balance due. Because he does not receive 100% of what he bills to his clients, Steve has learned that some clients have proved unworthy of that trust. However, as noted at the beginning of this chapter, he understands that it is rare for clinicians to receive 100% of the amount due to them, and after engaging in his best efforts to collect fees due him, he sees this as just a cost of doing business.

There are many avenues for clinicians to accept credit cards. Merchant accounts may be developed through local banks. Many computerized billing systems offer this as an option in their software. Some clinicians have developed credit card payment capabilities (two examples are found at http://www.professionalservices.com and http://www. therapypartner.com). Costs and procedures vary for each company. Clinicians are advised to explore all options and choose the one that works best for their practice situation. It is also important to sign the appropriate "Business Associate" agreement as per Health Insurance Portability and Accountability Act regulations. Be aware that when using an outside company, that company is your representative. Thus, the clinician could be held responsible for any misdeeds by the company. Although not an endorsement, one of the authors has used Professional Charges (http://www.professionalcharges.com) for several years. When a charge appears on the client's credit card statement, it does not include the clinician's name but rather ProfessionalCharges.com, which serves to protect the client's privacy.

Audits

By contractual agreement, an insurer or MCC has the right to audit your files to ensure that the billing that you have presented to them is accurate. Each contract should specify the audit process and your rights and responsibilities as a provider. It is especially important to be familiar with the appeals process should you disagree with the results of the audit.

The key in retaining all of the funds that have been provided to you by the insurance company following an audit lies in having effective documentation. Each insurer has its own criteria for what constitutes a complete record. If you have provided a clinically effective session of psychotherapy, are audited, and the documentation is not up to the standards set forth by the insurer, you will be asked to return the fee. Therefore, it is important to remain current with the documentation requirements for each of the insurers with which you have a contractual relationship.

Special Billing Issues

There are two special circumstances for billing that merit brief discussion. The first is billing Medicare, and the second is billing for workers compensation claims.

Medicare is a unique billing entity. To see Medicare patients, one must apply to be a Medicare provider. However, if you do not want to accept the Medicare fee schedule and follow their regulations, you cannot simply say, "I don't accept Medicare, but I will see you for my regular psychotherapy fee." To do this, one has to "opt out" of Medicare by completing an affidavit and sending it to the appropriate Medicare address. If the clinician has not opted out, then clients may not be reimbursed by Medicare when they submit a superbill. There is a 2-year period before one can apply to be a Medicare provider again after opting out. After opting out, the clinician essentially acts as an out-of-network provider for Medicare patients. Jean Thoensen is owner of an online billing service for clinicians (http://www.psychbiller.com) and has written an excellent primer on Medicare participation (available at http://archive.constantcontact.com/fs031/1101343307115/archive/110 2606343413.html).

Workers who have been injured on the job and are experiencing a mental health issue related to that injury may be eligible to have their mental health services paid for through the workers compensation system set in place by their state department of labor. Rules; regulations; eligibility; and how claims are opened, closed, and administered vary from state to state. Mental health treatment is usually authorized and monitored by a third party, and the clinician may contract with this third party to provide such services. However, it is important to understand all of the policies and procedures as they relate to the provision of care and for billing. For example, in most states, workers compensation is an *open system,* which means that clients do not retain privacy or privilege of communication as they would in a traditional psychotherapy setting. Most states require that treatment records be included with any submission of insurance forms. These records can be shared with the employer if the claims manager thinks it relevant, and the client cannot prevent this from happening. This can be of special concern to the client if the work-related injury is being disputed or a settlement amount is being developed. In the informed-consent process, it is essential that the client understand that the same privacy rights offered to many other psychotherapy clients are not available to them if they want their employer to pay for their mental health care. Unless they are willing to pay out of pocket, injured workers find themselves in a catch-22 situation. That is, if they choose not to have mental health as part of their workers compensation claim, they may prefer to use their regular health insurance (in which they would retain privacy) However, Box 10-a on the CMS-1500 asks whether the diagnosis being treated is related to an on-the-job injury. If so, the health insurer would want the workers compensation insurance company to pay for the mental health care.

Conclusion

To have a financially successful private practice, clinicians must set systems in place to collect fees routinely and effectively. We have emphasized the importance of a thoughtful and detail-oriented approach to the task to maximize collections and minimize outstanding balances due. Billing and collecting procedures also intersect with matters of ethics and law that must be carefully considered by clinicians to meet ethical and legal standards. Because of this, we think it essential for clinicians to follow these guidelines:

- Collect all fees due on the day of service, including applicable co-pays and deductibles.

- Maintain accurate and comprehensive treatment and financial records.
- Review insurance benefits with the client and verify their understanding of their responsibilities in the billing and collection process.
- Verify insurance benefits and obtain necessary preauthorizations before providing treatment.
- Carefully complete insurance claim forms and submit them expeditiously.
- Carefully review payment statements from insurance companies, and if they show that mistakes were made, request, in writing, corrections to them in a timely manner.
- Bill secondary insurance, if applicable.
- Understand that co-pays or deductibles due cannot be routinely waived and that all cases in which they are waived should be documented in the client's record.
- Accept credit cards to both increase collections and avoid a large balance due being built up.
- Understand that unique billing circumstances exist (e.g., workers compensation, Medicare) and become familiar with what is required in these alternative systems.
- Establish procedures to be prepared to pass a potential audit with flying colors.

Do It Yourself or Contract Out
The Pros and Cons of Using a Billing Service

5

A s has been mentioned, when the clinician has a fee-for-service practice, the billing and collecting are typically easy. Clients write a check or pay by credit card or cash at each session. If clients would like to be reimbursed by an insurance company, the clinician provides them with a superbill receipt that they may submit on their own behalf. Such arrangements are clearly and easily addressed in the informed financial agreement at the outset of the professional relationship and are typically implemented in a straightforward manner.

However, when the clinician bills an insurance company for reimbursement, the task is one that can take significant time, energy, and financial resources. Clinicians must decide whether they will take sole responsibility for this task, delegate it to an employee, or outsource it to a company specializing in this area. Each of these choices has different costs, and a decision must be made as to which resources will be expended toward this important business function. Essentially, we must collect the fees owed to us if we are to maintain a successful or even viable business. Thus, how one ensures that all fees owed are collected in a timely manner is a vital function in the business of practice.

Recently, we posed the following question to clinicians on two e-mail discussion lists:

In the scenario in which one bills insurance (that is, not a fee-for-service practice), one must make a choice about how best to bill and collect from clients. We would appreciate hearing what people think about doing the billing yourself (or having it done by a staff member within your practice whom you supervise) versus contracting with an outside billing service.

On the basis of the responses received, it appears the decision is related to personal values about time, the willingness to take on a tedious task and be educated about changes in billing regulations and insurance law, the need for control, and tolerance of others' mistakes. These are discussed in the sections following the basic description of billing services and opportunities for doing billing on one's own.

Billing Services

Enter the key words *mental health billing service* into an Internet search engine, and numerous hits will emerge of companies who provide this service. With the ubiquity of electronic communication, these companies are able to serve clinicians across the nation without being physically located in their local area.

Billing services provide a wide array of services. The extent of services provided typically depends on which services the clinician wishes to purchase. The more you purchase, the higher the cost. One billing service found through an Internet search indicated that it offers a "Gold Service Plan, a Diamond Service Plan, and a Platinum Service Plan." Hunt (2005) pointed out that billing services can be expensive—they can charge between 7% and 10% of monies collected. Typical services offered include the following: client insurance benefits verification and client financial consultation, obtaining initial insurance preauthorization, advising the clinician of clients' financial obligations and authorization limitations, electronic filing of claims, producing and mailing monthly statements to clients if a balance is due, producing monthly reports showing all postings (including charges, payments, and write-offs), and conducting bimonthly account status reviews.

As can be seen from the list of typical services provided by billing companies, there is much to keep track of in billing and collecting. If this is not your forte or inclination, then you may forget to bill sessions or bill in an untimely manner, so that the required filing deadline (usually 60–90 days for most insurance companies) passes. No fees are collected in these circumstances, and the client cannot then be asked to pay for your error. If this happens frequently, then the money saved by someone else competently collecting on your behalf may indeed pay for itself or earn you more than you might collect on your own.

Jean Thoenson, owner of Psychbiller, LLC (http://www.psychbiller. com/), has presented 10 pieces of advice for the clinician to consider when choosing a billing service (described in Walfish & Barnett, 2008). Some of these include the following:

- Ensure that the business is licensed and registered. This business will be a covered entity under the Health Insurance Portability and Accountability Act and will be collecting on your behalf. Therefore, you need to make sure you are dealing with a legitimate, and not fly-by-night, business.
- Ensure that the business has significant experience in mental health billing. Experience in billing for physicians may not transfer to billing for mental health services because of the insurance companies and managed care organizations having different requirements.
- Obtain several references from customers of billing services before making a decision on which to use.
- Have a specific contract that spells out the responsibilities of each party. Will the company verify insurance benefits for each client? The charges for each service provided (e.g., insurance verification, billing, generation of reports, time to review accounts) need to be specifically delineated.
- Know how the claims are submitted (paper vs. electronically) and how often (daily, weekly, monthly).

Hunt (2005) also advised visiting the billing service, if possible, and examining sample bills and reports. If they are not in your local area, we urge an initial telephone conversation to address your questions and concerns.

Even with the billing service doing most of the work, there are details that the clinician must pay attention to if collections are to be optimized. The billing service needs to know whom to bill, the service provided, the amount charged, and any co-pays that were collected on the date of service. Therefore, clinicians must fill out sheets (either on paper and faxed or online) with each client's identifying information and insurance company and daily logs that indicate which services were provided, along with the charges for each. In addition, and most important, clinicians must routinely confirm that the billing service is doing its job properly. If billed charges are not paid in a timely manner, is the insurance company contacted? If payment is denied, does the clinician find out why and intervene or appeal the decision? It is also important for clinicians to know whether clients are not paying their bill and running up a large balance that could result in the clinician being placed in an ethical dilemma (i.e., the client clinically needing services but not paying for them). Nonpayment of fees can be conceptualized as both a business and a clinical issue. Therefore, it is important for the clinician to review reports of balances due routinely.

Thoensen (as described in Walfish & Barnett, 2008) also noted some potential downsides of using an external billing service. First, your account may be one of numerous accounts that the company manages. Although services are paid by the percentage of monies collected and an incentive exists to recover as much as possible, to the billing service, you may be just another account. Neither of us uses a billing service, and each long ago decided, on the basis of negative experiences, that "no one collects money for me like I collect money for me." Second, as your agent, the company is an extension of you and your practice. Therefore, any ethical breaches or illegal behavior on the part of your agent become your responsibility. Third, if for any reason you are unhappy with the services received and wish to switch to another billing service, there may be a financial disincentive to do so; most companies have a one-time setup charge for taking on new accounts, and most do not indicate on their website the fee charged for this. It is important to find out all costs related to beginning and ending a relationship with a billing service before entering into a contract.

Billing services make mistakes. Insurance companies make mistakes. It is important for clinicians to understand that even though someone may be billing on their behalf, it is essential that all billing and collecting be closely monitored. When mistakes are made, it is also important to clarify whether it will be the billing service or the private practitioner who will follow up to correct the mistake.

Billing On Your Own

The development of billing software has allowed clinicians to do their own billing. However, this requires a significant commitment of time and energy, as well as a modest financial investment. The extent may depend on whether you wish to provide yourself with the "gold," "silver," or "platinum" approaches to billing and collecting. If you bill on your own, it means that you may be verifying insurance benefits; advising clients about their benefits (including co-pays and plan limitations); submitting claim forms; entering financial data for payments received; generating statements of balances due and mailing them out to clients; and generating summary reports to track amount of income, receivables owed, and sources from where your revenue is coming.

Most insurance companies will allow you to verify insurance benefits online. However, some services will require preauthorization. For example, to preauthorize psychological testing for his presurgical psychological evaluations before his client's weight loss surgery, Steve Walfish is often required to speak with a case manager at a managed care company. Often, this is smooth and easy and requires only 5 minutes. However, there have been times when it has taken 30 to 45 minutes because he was placed on hold for 10 minutes, only to learn that he was calling the wrong precertification center. This resulted in being switched to another call center and being placed on hold or occasionally being cut off and having to start the process from the beginning. Then, the person on the other end of the phone occasionally has not understood why psychological testing was necessary for someone with a medical diagnosis. To say the least, these are frustrating experiences.

On his website (http://www.assessmentpsychology.com/), in the section "Billing and Practice Management Software for Psychologists and Mental Health Practitioners," William Benet presents a list of commercially available software programs for billing and practice management, along with a link to each company's website. This is a good starting point for finding the right package. However, software programs are constantly in development, so it is best to do an Internet search on the key words *mental health billing software.* It also likely will be helpful to consult with colleagues about the billing systems they use and to find out whether they are satisfied with the program itself and with the customer service assistance that is available for training, to answer questions, or to fix problems.

Many programs offer simple billing programs. Others offer features that may be purchased as an upgrade to include a scheduling program, as well as a clinical record program. These integrated programs save the clinician time and centralize all relevant information. However, the more features desired, the higher the purchasing price. It is important not simply to buy the "biggest and best" because it is the most expensive but to see how the program will actually fit into your practice routine and meet your specific needs. That is, if you are not going to keep an electronic schedule, there is no reason to purchase such a feature.

Costs of software systems vary. Choosing three programs as examples on the day of this writing, the website-advertised cost of a solo practitioner program through TheraQuick is $795, through ShrinkRapt is $595, and through Confidant is $289. Cost for a solo practitioner package is less than a multiple-user package. It is important to determine whether there are additional costs for training or customer service. In addition, most systems have an annual upgrade and customer service charge, so it is also important to be aware of these costs because you are likely to use the system for a long time. Switching billing systems is an annoying task because the old and new systems do not integrate, and all client information must be entered manually into the new system. We have known large group practices to be dissatisfied with their billing system but found it too daunting to move to a new system because data would have to be transferred for more than 1,000 clients. As such, they decided to continue with their existing system even though they were unhappy with its performance. Most systems have demonstration programs that can be downloaded. We encourage you to use this feature and test run several to see which will be best for your practice.

Billing through these programs is relatively easy and does not require a great time investment. On a one-time basis, you must enter your practice information (e.g., name, address, tax ID number, National Provider Identifier number), the types of services that you might provide (e.g., initial evaluation, individual psychotherapy, family psychotherapy, psychological testing), and the fee charged for each service. This information is stored in the program's memory. Then, for all clients, on a one-time basis, you must enter their identifying information, the name of their insurance company, and their unique insurance policy number. This is the basic information that would appear on a standard CMS-1500 form. The programs store the insurance companies and their addresses, so this information does not have to be entered each time. For example, the first time a client who has Cigna insurance is entered into the system, this information is entered into the program's memory. Then all it takes is a simple click on "Cigna insurance" for each subsequent client with the same insurance company. Then, to bill for each visit, you enter the date of service and simply click on the type of service. Once you are up and running, this process takes about 30 seconds. You can decide how often to bill (e.g., after each session, once per month) for these sessions.

Most of these programs provide the opportunity to bill either electronically or with a paper claim. With paper claims, you must purchase the CMS-1500 forms (at a local office supply store or a company found on the Internet), print out the billing statements, place postage on each envelope, and mail them. With electronic claims you enter a code for the insurance company and click on a link. In addition to saving money, electronic billing usually is processed more quickly by the insurance company.

Submitting claims electronically is not time-consuming, but it is time-consuming to enter data into the billing system regarding client co-pays, insurance payments received, and write-offs that may be in effect for that particular payor. For example, if you charge $100 per session, the amount that will be allowed for that session will differ for United Behavioral Health, Magellan, Tricare, Value Options, Cigna, and your local Blue Cross plan. So, to calculate whether the client has a balance due, this information must be entered into the program's database.

Another time-consuming task is sending out balance-due statements after receiving payments from the insurance company. If everything goes as expected, there should be no balance due because the client has paid his or her co-pay and the insurance company has paid its expected portion. However, sometimes insurance companies do not pay the expected portion because deductibles are not met, the portion expected is incorrect, or benefits are unexpectedly exhausted. These statements must be generated, mailed out, and then entered into the system once payment has been received. If payment is not received, a follow-up statement must be sent to the client, or if agreed-on ahead of time, a credit card will be billed for the amount due.

Free Online Billing

Many insurance and managed care companies allow the private practitioner to bill for sessions on the company's web portal at no charge. Indeed, they prefer that billing be done in this manner because they view it as most cost-effective. Advantages to the clinician of such an arrangement are that it is an easy format to bill, there is no charge for billing, payment is received faster than with a paper claim, and there is quick feedback as to whether the client has exhausted the authorized number of sessions because the claim will be rejected quickly if this is the case.

Another option is to use one of the free online billing services that have emerged. An example of one such service is Office Ally (http://www.officeally.com). Essentially, these services act as a clearinghouse for claims submissions for the insurance companies. Office Ally's website explains that it is paid for each transaction by the insurance company and in turn chooses not to turn around and bill the clinician for submitting the claim. This company also offers value-added services that do have fees associated with them. Other clearinghouse companies charge the clinician as well as the insurer. These companies may be found by entering the key words *insurance billing clearinghouses* into an Internet search engine.

It is important to note that these free online mechanisms to bill insurance companies for services rendered are not equivalent to having a billing software system. The clinician must develop a system, either through purchasing a billing software program or using a simple spread sheet, to keep track of what has been billed and collected for each client as well as the sources of income (e.g., referral source, insurance company).

This important bookkeeping function is essential for the small business owner so that he or she can understand, analyze, and act on financial data to optimize success in practice (Walfish & Barnett, 2008).

Factors to Consider When Making a Decision

It is important to make a personal decision about the cost-effectiveness of using a billing service. Clinicians with full-time practices may find their time better spent treating clients and thus creating income. These clinicians may find the expenses incurred by using a billing service well worth the cost. Additionally, the larger one's practice (whether an individual or group practice), the more data one must manage and the more meticulous one must be. For those with part-time practices, it may be more time- and cost-efficient to manage one's own billing and collecting, especially when they take into account the one-time setup fee charged by billing services. Those with the time and inclination may be better served by doing these activities themselves.

As noted earlier, we asked clinicians to provide us with opinions regarding their decision to hire a billing service or to take responsibility for this task. As you can see from the following quotes from these clinicians, the underlying reasons for making these decisions are idiosyncratic. These categories are not independent of each other, and naturally there is some overlap that may be found across the general categories.

VALUE PLACED ON TIME

I used to be a do-it-myselfer. This is how I kept my overhead low. However, time is now more valuable to me than money.

I have outsourced billing for at least 20 years and would never bring it in house. I think that they know the ins and outs of billing to a greater extent than I, and they attend the webinars and Medicare training sessions. They are then responsible for updating software and hardware, a cost I don't have to incur. I am then free to see more patients or have time to relax.

We have always used a billing company mostly because I have no idea how to do the billing and am too busy to learn.

The way that I look at the expense of a billing service is to compare how many psychotherapy hours a month I "pay" for the service. For me, that is under 5 clinical hours. I would much rather do another 5 hours of psychotherapy per month rather than bill and follow up with billing errors or other confusion.

NEED FOR CONTROL

To get paid with third party reimbursement, one must: assemble required information to complete a CMS-1500 form, provide data for each service and billing unit, know where to send it, send it, follow up to make sure it gets paid and paid correctly, it still needs to be entered on a patient ledger to credit the payment, and if denied, ignored, or paid incorrectly, it has to be followed up—maybe several times. My perspective is that a billing company will not reliably do all of these steps, in which case, there will be a lot of earned money that will never be seen. If done in house, it needs to be done correctly and systematically to collect all you are entitled to. From a business perspective, you have more control over it in house.

I can't for the life of me figure out why clinicians use a billing service other than that they're afraid to tackle it themselves. But these services are a huge time and money drain, and make constant mistakes they don't catch themselves.

I have a billing person (accounts manager). She has her own office and bills only in accord with what I provide; she makes no independent decisions. All payments come directly to me, and I provide her with a list of payments received. I have heard some horror stories of psychologists who trust their billing personnel and have been ripped off.

TOLERANCE FOR MISTAKES OF OTHERS

I tried using someone that a colleague had recommended for billing who was beginning her own billing practice. It was a disaster. I never had a handle on what was happening, found multiple errors, and actually got payments later for three patients that were not mine!!! These then had to be voided and returned to the insurance company. Therefore, I do my own billing again and just deal with it.

WILLINGNESS TO TAKE ON A TEDIOUS AND LABORIOUS TASK

I have used several billing services in the past, done billing myself, and now use the services of my husband as an independent contractor for billing. When I did it myself, I found myself getting overwhelmed with the minutia of coding, electronic claims, and clearinghouses and spent a lot of time on details that I really didn't care about but needed to care about to get paid.

You spend a few bucks but don't have to spend your time dealing with headaches, billing secondary insurance, learning the software, etc. For me it is one less detail I have to deal with when the billing service does that piece.

I have never done my own billing. I have absolutely no interest, and probably less skill than interest. My current service does more than billing, including verification of benefits, dealing with tricky insurance claims, dogging insurance companies for nonpayment, primary and secondary billing, as well as generating monthly statements for clients as well as monthly reports for me. I have also found that having my service verify benefits in advance has decreased confusion over coverage to practically zero.

Conclusion

In this chapter, we have outlined two methods for billing insurance: outsourcing the task to a billing service or doing it yourself (personally or through office support staff). There are plusses and minuses to each of these options, and clearly no one size fits all. Potential plusses of using a billing service are the following:

- You can use an experienced business specializing in billing for mental health services.
- You save time.
- You can subcontract a tedious task.
- Your billing and collecting will be organized by someone else (this is especially beneficial if you are a disorganized person).
- You can delegate queries about billing from clients to the billing service.

Potential minuses of using a billing service are the following:

- The cost can be significant.
- You have to turn over control of your finances to a third party.
- You may not receive optimal attention because you will be one of multiple accounts.
- There may be a financial penalty for leaving the service.
- There will be new start-up costs if you move to another company.
- Significant time will be spent monitoring the company if it makes many mistakes.
- You are responsible for any ethical or legal lapses of the billing service.

Potential plusses of billing on your own are the following:

- You save money on billing costs.
- You have total control over billing and collections.

Potential minuses of billing on your own are:

- You may spend a significant amount of time on billing and collecting.
- Dealing with insurance companies can be frustrating.

Clinicians are urged to look at their own practice situation and examine their own values and beliefs about time and money, need for control, tolerance for mistakes of others, and the willingness to take on a tedious task in coming to a decision that appears to be the best choice for them.

Billing and Collecting for Forensic Mental Health Services | 6

H
ess (2006b) noted the prodigious growth in the collaboration between law and psychology. One aspect of this growth has been the application of psychology in legal settings. Mental health clinicians have always played a role in both the civil and criminal components in our justice system. For example, in civil cases, clinicians may evaluate a litigant to determine the presence and extent of any emotional injuries due to a specific event, such as a motor vehicle accident (Walfish, 2006), or complete a child custody evaluation with recommendations for parenting plans. In criminal cases, clinicians may serve the court by helping to determine a defendant's competency to stand trial, assess if mitigating circumstances may have been present in the commission of a crime to aid in sentencing, or evaluate a defendant to determine whether a deferred prosecution is appropriate pending treatment for a condition that may have been related to the commission of a crime.

In recent years, there has been an increase in the number of clinicians who include forensic work in their practice. Indeed, some do only forensic work. There are multiple reasons for this increase. First is the greater recognition of how clinicians can help the key players in the judicial system: judges and attorneys. Clinicians can provide judges with objective opinions so that they can come to better decisions.

Clinicians can provide attorneys with objective data and opinions to help them be better advocates for their clients. Second, clinicians have sought alternative ways to practice that do not fall under of the purview of insurance and managed care (Walfish, 2010). Indeed, in two surveys of how private practice psychologists earn a living outside of managed care, forensic psychology activities was the category most often mentioned. This included 37 practice activities in the first survey (Walfish, 2001) and 38 in the second survey (Le & Walfish, 2007). Because forensic work is not considered medical in nature, health insurance is not a consideration. Third, fees for forensic work tend to be higher than traditional clinical services. Hess (1998) cited forensic practice to be among the most lucrative of specialties within psychology, possibly surpassed only by neuropsychological assessment.

Because this is an area of increased participation by mental health clinicians, it is important to understand the specialized billing and collection procedures and their ethical implications. The rules governing clinical practice in one's office conducting individual psychotherapy do not specifically generalize to practice in the forensic arena. In this chapter, we discuss billing for forensic mental health services. Specifically, we discuss issues related to ethics documents, financial concerns in terms of both informed consent and the setting of fees, understanding what is being reimbursed, how to get paid for services provided, when to get paid, and the importance of avoiding contingency fees.

Ethics Documents

Clinicians practicing in the area of forensics must become familiar with two important documents before ever accepting a case. The first is the American Psychology–Law Society's "Specialty Guidelines for Forensic Psychology" (Committee on the Revision of Specialty Guidelines for Forensic Psychology, 2008; available at http://www.ap-ls.org/about psychlaw/92908sgfp.pdf). Section 7 of this document focuses on fees, specifically determining fees and fee arrangements. Section 8 focuses on issues of informed consent.

The second is the American Psychological Association's "Guidelines for Child Custody Evaluations in Family Law Proceedings" (American Psychological Association, 2010b) for those doing custody work (available at http://www.apa.org/practice/guidelines/child-custody.pdf). These guidelines share implications for informed consent and the determination of fee agreements. We are unaware of any specialty guidelines for forensic work that have been developed by the other mental health professions.

Informed Consent About Fees

As with psychotherapy clients, when providing forensic services it is important to clarify all aspects of the professional relationship and services offered at the very beginning. This may include, but is not limited to, identifying the client (e.g., the person who comes to your office, the guardian ad litem, the court), the exact questions being addressed in the evaluation, the questions not to be addressed in the consultation, the way the results of the evaluation will be communicated to include sharing them with others, and payment arrangements.

Hess (1998) discussed ethical and professional considerations in accepting forensic referrals. He highlighted the importance of understanding and framing the consultation from the outset of the professional relationship, because this may set the stage for how the case will proceed over the long term. Blau (1998) advocated discussing fee arrangements during the first phone call when either an attorney or a client asks the clinician to become involved in the case. He stressed the importance of the expert outlining all fees involved and what time and services will be charged for, then ensuring that this arrangement is agreeable to the person retaining the expert.

For example, most forensic evaluators will have either an hourly or a predetermined flat fee for completing their evaluation. However, charges for involvement in forensic cases do not stop there. Other services that may be billed include the production of a report summarizing the findings (if desired), consultation with the attorney regarding the findings, time spent reviewing case materials in preparation for deposition or court testimony, time spent with the attorney discussing questions that may be posed during direct examination and cross-examination, travel time to and from a courtroom appearance, time spent in deposition or on the witness stand, and time spent waiting to testify. At times, the expert may need to do specialized research to be a better witness. The amount of preparation time and the amount of time spent conducting research should be estimated by the expert and communicated to the parties (e.g., retaining attorney or the client) so those paying the fees can make an informed decision in retaining the expert. Knapp and VandeCreek (2001) noted the importance of informing attorneys or clients of the possibility they may need to seek additional consultation from other clinicians and the costs involved in such consultation.

Woody (1998) presented multiple ways that a clinician can incur the wrath of an attorney. One is to charge an excessive amount for preparing for a deposition or a court appearance. Woody opined, "When a psychologist submits a bill for an exorbitant amount of time allegedly spent on reviewing records, a legal firestorm is likely to result" (p. 11). Some cases are complex, and there are boxes of records. Other cases are routine and do not contain a lot of external records as part of the case file. If a case file contains 25 to 50 pages and the expert bills for 5 to 10 hours of record review, the person retaining the expert may indeed have sticker shock when he or she receives the bill for services. Similarly, if research is needed on a case and the expert bills for 10 hours of research, the retaining attorney may wonder whether the person was really an "expert" in the first place. Woody (1998), who is both a psychologist and an attorney, pointed out that when attorneys become angry at a clinician's perceived overbilling, they may want to teach the expert a lesson:

> One "teaching technique" favored by some attorneys is to file a motion for an order of contempt and financial sanctions (which would require the psychologist to pay the expenses incurred by the attorney in seeking the court order). Even if the court does not grant the motion, such a technique can potentially damage one's reputation, increase stress and anxiety, and require the psychologist to pay for personal legal representation. (p. 12)

It is important that the mental health clinician develop a written financial agreement that clarifies all payment arrangements from the outset. With this agreement there are no surprises for the person receiving the bill or questions about whether the clinician should be receiving payment for the services rendered. A sample forensic agreement may be found on the website of the American Psychological Association Insurance Trust (http://www.apait.org/apait/download.aspx). In addition, many clinicians provide a copy of their agreements on their websites. Entering the terms *forensic psychology agreement* into an Internet search will yield many such documents for review.

Setting Fees

Clinicians working in a forensic context may be paid by the court, the attorney requesting their expert services, or an individual who is involved in a court case. Each of these may have different implications for fees earned for services provided.

Melton, Petrila, Poythress, and Slobogin (1997) noted that in evaluations for the court, the government has a set fee schedule. For example, they may pay x dollars to complete an examination to determine whether a defendant is competent to stand trial. They may pay y dollars to complete a psychological evaluation to aid in sentencing in a juvenile court case. They may pay z dollars to complete a drug and alcohol evaluation for someone convicted of a crime in which substance abuse may have been a mitigating factor. These fees tend to be set with little flexibility for negotiation.

Similar to the court, organizations may pay clinicians and have a set fee schedule. These typically leave little room for negotiation, although a psychologist colleague related the following story:

> I was asked by the Children's Aid Society to do an assessment for a legal case that would have to be done at Legal Aid rates. I didn't mind because my main source of income was from my job with the university, so I could afford to work for less. This was many years ago and they said the going rate for psychologists was $90 per hour. Out of curiosity I asked what they paid psychiatrists and was told $95 per hour. I told them if they valued psychiatrists more than psychologists they should get one to do the assessment. They said that they specifically wanted a psychologist for the particular case. I told them I would do it for the same rate as the psychiatrist, but they said the rates could not be changed. As I did not really need the business, I told them to get back to me if and when they paid the same rate as a psychiatrist. They called me a week later and had changed the fee schedule.

When negotiation for fees is possible, negotiate from a position of strength (Walfish & Barnett, 2008). This strength is typically found in the ability to say "no thank you" to the referral.

When being hired by a defense or plaintiff's attorney or an individual requesting an evaluation (e.g., for a child custody evaluation), clinicians can set their own fee schedule. It is up to the individuals hiring the expert to determine whether they are willing to pay these fees. The fees charged are not dependent on one's professional discipline. That is, psychiatrists, psychologists, clinical social workers, counselors, and marriage and family therapists can all charge the same fee for completing the forensic work. For example, we are aware of a clinical social worker who charges $500 per hour for her specialized evaluations. The attorneys hiring her do not balk at her fee because the data that she can gather in her specialty area and the testimony that she can provide in personal injury cases can result in six-figure (and at times seven-figure) settlement awards for their clients. She routinely turns away cases because the demand for her services is greater than she can provide.

There are differences of opinion as to whether fees for forensic services should be similar to or different from fees charged for traditional office clinical services. For example, Bennett et al. (2006) indicated that many psychologists charge more than their regular fee schedule for the stress involved in forensic work. Zuckerman (2008) suggested that fees for forensic services are commonly billed at twice the normal office rate. In contrast, Blau (1998) argued that office and forensic fees should be identical. He suggested that if they are dissimilar, the clinician may be accused of bias on cross-examination and only providing testimony as a way to increase income. Woody (1998) viewed inflating forensic fees above normal office fees as one way to incur the wrath of an attorney. When it comes to billing for forensic fees, Melton et al. (1997) noted,

> Our experience is that forensic practitioners are far from uniform in their billing practices. Many charge rates that are higher than for clinical services. Some charge more for time in deposition or in court than evaluation services that take place out of court. The bottom-line amount a client is willing to pay may also influence a clinician's willingness to accept a case. None of these approaches is necessarily inappropriate. (p. 110)

We believe that it is reasonable to charge higher fees for forensic work, especially if depositions or court appearances may be part of the case. However, Blau's (1998) and Woody's (1998) warnings should be heeded, and the clinician should have an adequate answer to any challenge of this practice. Depositions and court appearances can be disruptive to clinicians' practices. They may need to be on call to make their appearance; lengths of trials are unpredictable, expected testimony time can be postponed, and regular psychotherapy clients may have to be rescheduled.

What Are You Being Paid For?

While testifying in a divorce case related to the possibility that a husband might have a substance abuse problem, the following exchange took place between Steve Walfish (SW) and the husband's attorney:

Attorney: Dr. Walfish, how much are you being paid for your testimony?

SW: I'm not being paid for my testimony.

Attorney: But you have prepared for court today, reviewed documents, come to a conclusion and traveled to court today, so once again I will ask you, can you please tell me how much you are being paid for your testimony?

SW: Once again, I repeat I am not being paid for my testimony.

Attorney: So you are not being paid at all to be here today?

SW: No Ma'am. I am being paid to be here to answer whatever questions you may have for me related to this case.

Naturally, the attorney knew this was the case but was hoping Steve would say, "I'm being paid $1,000 for my testimony" and then could advocate that he was just a "hired gun" and have the opinion disqualified as being biased.

Mart (2006) stated that the role of the clinician in forensic practice is one of objectivity. It is essential that anyone doing this work strive to be as unbiased as possible, regardless of who is paying the expert's fees. Mart pointed out that the American Psychological Association Ethics

Code and the Committee on the Revision of Specialty Guidelines for Forensic Psychology (2008) urge clinicians to avoid relationships that might create bias in the professional opinion rendered. He asserted, "If you find, by a remarkable coincidence your conclusions always support the position of the person that retained you, then you need to take a hard look at your objectivity" (p. 112). The objectivity of mental health experts doing forensic work has long been called into question (Hagen, 1997). LaFortune and Carpenter (1998) surveyed child custody evaluators and found that "providing an accurate and fair picture and to be unbiased as the most desirable characteristics of a child custody expert" (p. 213). For this reason, these child custody evaluators preferred an employment arrangement in which both of the litigants were responsible for the costs of their services. When this is not feasible (e.g., because one of the parties has access to a disproportionate amount of money compared with the other party), it is still essential that the clinician remain objective in coming to conclusions and making recommendations to the court.

The clinician is typically being retained to provide an "expert opinion." At times attorneys may try and have the clinician designated as a "fact witness" instead of an "expert witness." Bennett et al. (2006) elaborated that "what distinguishes expert witnesses from fact witnesses is that the expert witness has relevant specialized knowledge beyond that of the average person. This knowledge may qualify them to provide opinions as well as facts" (p. 134). If one is a fact witness, there is no special reason to pay the clinician any additional fees other than a standard witness fee. It is important to have this clarified at the outset of the request to appear. If the attorney insists, it may be important to ask the judge in the case to render an opinion before testifying. Woody (1994) noted, "If a psychologist is paid as a fact witness they have to appear and state facts (e.g., dates of service, payments made, verification of records), but there is no duty to render an expert opinion per se" (p. 18). However, Woody also warned that a judge may have a negative reaction if the clinician is asked questions as an expert but declines to answer because he or she has only been asked to appear in court as a fact witness. Thus, if possible, one's role should be clarified from the outset, and definitely before giving testimony.

Forensic cases can be complex and time-consuming. They can involve review of relevant records and conducting the assessment, which will include a clinical interview and perhaps also psychometric testing. Record review can range anywhere from a few pages to a few boxes of material. When there is a large amount to review, it is important to have a discussion with the referring attorney regarding what to review and what not to review. If several boxes need to be reviewed, it is important to estimate how much time this will take because this can easily add up to a significant invoice. There may be a need to conduct interviews with collaterals who can shed light on the person being evaluated. In the case of child custody evaluations, there is a need to observe each parent inter-acting with the child (or children) as well as to gather information from other individuals such as other family members, neighbors, teachers, and the like. A written report may also need to be produced. Forensic reports can range in length from a few pages to hundreds of pages, depending on the preferred reporting style of the clinician and the needs of the case. Time may be spent discussing the results of the case informally with attorneys or more formally in deposition as well as driving to court, waiting to testify, testifying, and driving back to your office following the hearing. All of these activities may be billed for in forensic cases.

Getting Paid for Your Services

Most attorneys are honorable, and there would never be a question as to whether payment will be received for services rendered. However, Melton et al. (1997) stated, "Law firms have been known not to pay their experts, especially when the experts opinions are not particularly useful" (p. 111). Hess (2006a) related the following experience:

> In a pair of related cases, the attorneys were not known for their integrity, and the psychologist had an understanding that they would bill when the cases were concluded. The two attorneys kept telling the psychologist, who had provided the case reviews and reports, that the psychologist would soon be called for the next hearing. They never informed the psychologist when the cases and appeals were exhausted. More than a year later, the psychologist found out in the *Law Reporter* that the appeal was lost. The attorneys had little incentive to call the psychologist because they would be paying the fee from their pocket, not from a client's award. (p. 678)

Eventually the psychologist was paid for these cases, but only through diligence and persistence.

It is important to clarify in writing the fees that will be charged, who will be responsible for paying them, and when they are due. In some cases, it will be the attorney, who will then pass along these costs to his or her client. For example, Steve Walfish completed a psychological evaluation with a client following a motor vehicle accident. As per their written financial agreement, the attorney wrote Steve a check immediately on receipt of the report and an invoice.

To highlight the need for a written financial agreement before com-pleting the work, consider the experience of this psychologist colleague:

> I received a referral from a criminal defense attorney in solo private law practice. The attorney asked me to provide an evaluation with one of his clients for sentencing purposes. I

explained my practice procedures, including my payment arrangements, on which we both orally agreed. I did not ask for a retainer since we had come to an agreement. Several months passed after I sent the report and invoice, with no payment received. I sent a second notice. Then I received a phone call from the attorney who said the client would send me a check. I reminded the attorney [that he] had agreed to pay me directly. He agreed to send me a check. No check arrived, and two months later I left the attorney a voicemail. He returned the call along with an argument that he could not comingle funds and therefore it would be inappropriate for the attorney to pay me directly. Not having an understanding of comingling funds I acquiesced and decided to let the matter drop. Afterwards, I looked up the concept of commingling funds and knew he could have paid me. Due to the high-profile nature of the attorney, I did not pursue the matter further. I still have not been paid, but I lose no sleep at night because I will not take another referral from this attorney without a hefty retainer.

Here is another example of attorney misbehavior, but from a psychologist who did not let the matter lie:

A workers compensation (WC) case was accepted for treatment. The patient had agreed to be responsible for all fees, irrespective of WC, but I agreed to defer payment, pending settlement of the case. The case was settled, and all fees were paid directly to the attorney. The attorney initially stalled on payment, then ignored requests for payment. We discussed with the patient his responsibility for obtaining payment, and this resulted in the attorney starting to return our calls and acknowledging that the patient had contacted him regarding this and more promises of payment. After warning the attorney that nonpayment would result in an ethics complaint, I filed a complaint with the state board regulating attorneys. This resulted in a flurry of activity, apologies, and finally payment in full.

When to Get Paid?

As can be seen from these examples, forensic clinicians must set a system in place to ensure they are paid for their services. It is especially important to be paid for your services before rendering an expert opinion or producing a written report.

In child custody cases, it is important to get a retainer at the beginning of the case. Some evaluators charge a flat fee for the evaluation, whereas others charge an hourly rate. When charging an hourly rate, the fees can build quickly. If and when this retainer appears to be drained, it is essential that the evaluator ask for further monies before continuing work on the case. If one member of the couple does not like how things are going, then he or she may balk or delay paying further funds toward an evaluation that will not result in the desired outcome.

Once an opinion has been rendered, if the results are disappointing to a person responsible for paying the bill, he or she may have little incentive to make payment. Mart (2006) noted that when testifying in criminal cases, a person found guilty may be unavailable or have no interest in paying his or her bill. Furthermore, if the individual is simply interested in having your testimony on record, once that takes place, paying you may quickly become a low priority. Therefore, Mart advocated being paid before going to court or deposition. Each of us has often been handed checks at the beginning of a deposition or in the courthouse before testifying. If the clinician is not paid according to the agreement, he or she is still responsible to appear in court or at deposition and answer questions. Following the hearing, the clinician should seek payment and, as a last resort, ask the court to intervene.

Objectivity is paramount in providing expert witness opinions. Knapp and VandeCreek (2001) suggested that failure to be paid before testimony, or any other fee dispute, can serve to tarnish the objectivity of the expert witness. They cited an example of "covert bargaining" about fees when an attorney requested a subtle change in the expert's report (e.g., "I'll see what I can do about getting you paid"). Knapp and VandeCreek noted that the psychologist's failure to respond to this subtle influence resulted in the attorney's nonpayment.

There are cases in which clinicians provide ongoing consultation to an attorney on a case. This may include evaluation of a client, preparation of a client for court testimony, and trial strategy preparation. Blau (1998) noted the importance of not allowing bills to accumulate to large amounts. He presented a letter of agreement for use with the attorney for how fees will be paid, as well as a sample invoice that clinicians may use in forensic cases.

Avoid Contingency Payments

When he practiced in Washington State, Steve Walfish became interested in the research on the incidence of posttraumatic stress disorder (PTSD) following motor vehicle accidents (MVAs). He discovered that according to Blanchard, Hickling, Taylor, Loos, and Gerardi (1994), 46% of individuals who had been involved in an MVA and sought medical attention within 1 week could be diagnosed 1 to 4 months later with PTSD. On the basis of these data, Steve developed an evaluation service for individuals who had been in MVAs and received referrals from personal injury attorneys, chiropractors, and physicians (Walfish, 2006).

When Steve moved to Atlanta, he met with a large firm of attorneys who specialized in personal injury cases. In a conference room, he met with 10 attorneys who were enthusiastic about this service because they (a) were interested in having clients who needed mental health services receive them, and (b) they believed that if such a diagnosis were present, the financial settlement or jury award for their client would be greater. The attorneys indicated that they could easily send five to 10 clients per month for evaluation. However, this consultation never came to fruition because of disagreement over how the psychological services would be paid. Steve wanted a guarantee of payment from the attorneys for his services, regardless of the outcome of the case. The attorneys wanted Steve to be paid on a contingency basis, just as they were being paid. That is, payment for the mental health services would be rendered only if the case were won or settled in their client's favor. Their rationale was that they were taking a risk of only being paid if the case were won, so the psychologist should assume the same level of risk. Although the potential volume of referrals was significant, Steve turned down the consultation for ethical reasons to be discussed later in this chapter. The attorneys only shook their heads in disbelief that this much business was being turned away.

Although attorneys may get paid on a contingency basis, it is unethical for a clinician to be paid in this manner. Mart (2006) explained that being paid on a contingency basis may move the expert from a position of objectivity to one of advocate. He stated, "If you are only to be paid if your side wins the case this may influence the type of report that is written" (p. 162). Similarly, Knapp and VandeCreek (2001) indicated that contingency arrangements "give the appearance that psychologists could taint their testimony for their own financial gain" (p. 252).

Some clients may not have the funds to pay for an evaluation, and some attorneys do not like to make payments up front on behalf of their clients. It is ethical to wait for payment with a "Letter of Guarantee" (or "Letter of Protection") from the attorney that once the case has been completed they will be paid for their services. This Letter of Guarantee is most useful when it comes from attorneys and indicates that they will take responsibility for paying the expert's fee regardless of the outcome of the case. That is, even if their clients lose, the attorneys will pay the clinician. Many attorneys do not like to provide such a letter, preferring instead to have such a letter come from their client. That is, they do not want to take any financial risk. However, we caution against accepting such an arrangement. If clients guarantee the payment and do not receive a settlement, their incentive (or ability) to pay may be quite small. Woody (in press) presented a detailed discussion of Letters of Protection and ethical, as well as practical, aspects of this type of financial arrangement.

Two Closing Tidbits

Two other practice styles are worth mentioning because they relate to when the expert should be paid. First, Melton et al. (1997) cited the work of psychologist Stuart Greenberg, who asked for a nonrefundable retainer when he was asked to work on a case. There are some instances in which a clinician will be retained on a case and never asked to do any work. The attorney's purpose for such a tactic is to ensure that the other side will not retain the expert. Greenberg thought it important that he be reimbursed for his reputation and also because he might have "lost income" because he turned down other cases to make sure he had time to work on this case.

Second, when completing an evaluation for a flat fee, it is important to indicate in the financial agreement that the fee is nonrefundable. For example, Steve Walfish conducts substance abuse evaluations in divorce cases. There have been times when it was clear that the person had a substance abuse problem, and he or she became acutely aware that Steve knew this. In a few instances, they never completed the evaluation. They either argued for a change of evaluator or simply conceded they had a problem and went to treatment. If Steve never completed the evaluation, without such a clause in his agreement, he would not have been paid for his role in the evaluation because he did not complete a work product.

Conclusion

Billing for forensic mental health services carries a different set of policies, procedures, and ethical considerations than does billing for traditional psychotherapy services. It is essential that those practicing in a forensic context

- understand issues of informed consent in the forensic arena as opposed to traditional office practice,
- develop a strategy that one can defend in setting fees for forensic work,
- know exactly which professional service you are being paid to provide,
- remain objective in conducting evaluations and presenting findings and opinions,
- be paid before providing testimony to prevent ethical dilemmas from arising, and
- avoid being paid on a contingency basis.

Ethical Lapses by Clinicians in the Billing Process

7

R unning a busy practice can involve a wide range of activities that can more than occupy a clinician's time and attention. Such activities include preparing for and meeting with clients, consulting with colleagues, providing feedback on clients to referral sources, attending continuing education courses, keeping up with the professional literature, engaging in professional development activities, supervising staff, interacting with insurance companies, and conducting other billing and collection activities. Additionally, demands in the clinician's personal life may include relationship, health, financial, and other issues. Clinicians are not immune from experiencing stressful life events (Norcross & Guy, 2007; Rupert, Stevanovic, & Hunley, 2009), and an emphasis on adequate self-care may help to reduce ethical lapses or transgressions and should be viewed as an ethical imperative (Barnett, 2007).

In addition to coping with the challenges that all individuals face, clinicians must also effectively cope with those of being a psychotherapist or counselor and of providing clinical services in general. These may include working in isolation, working with chronic clients who do not improve or experience relapses, working with suicidal or violent clients, and administrative or bureaucratic demands such as documentation and paperwork requirements. Working with managed care and insurance companies presents challenges as well, such as coping with authorization denials, going through the appeals process, and difficulties collecting fees owed (Angerer, 2003; Barnett & Hillard, 2001; Rupert & Baird, 2004; Shinn, Rosario, Morch, & Chestnut, 1984). Taken together, all these challenges and stressors may have an impact on a clinician's ability to function effectively, competently, and ethically as a clinician.

This chapter discusses the most common causes of inaccurate billing and the most common types of ethical dilemmas that clinicians face in the billing process.

The Most Common Causes of Inaccurate Billing

Clinicians should be vigilant about a number of billing pitfalls. Clinicians experiencing significant financial pressures that result from participating in managed care and insurance may be tempted to bill for services that have not actually been provided. Examples may include meeting with clients for 30-minute sessions and billing as though 60-minute sessions were provided, meeting with a client weekly and billing as though the client was seen twice each week, treating a client in group psychotherapy and billing each group member as though individual psychotherapy were provided, having services provided by a supervisee such as an intern or student and billing as though the clinician provided the services, billing for services that never actually occurred, and billing for uncovered services (e.g., telephone calls, report writing, missed appointments) as though they were covered services such as psychotherapy sessions. Although readers may be saying to themselves, "Of course this shouldn't be done," these examples are based on actual practices reported by clinicians.

It is clear that all services provided should be billed accurately and that clinicians should not engage in dishonesty, fraud, or deception as is stated in the National Association of Social Workers (1999) Code of Ethics (Standard 4.04). Furthermore, the American Psychological Association (APA; 2010a) Ethics Code states clearly in Standard 6.06, Accuracy in Reports to Payors and Funding Sources,

> In their reports to payors for services . . . psychologists take reasonable steps to ensure the accurate reporting of the nature of the service provided . . . the fees, charges, or payments, and where applicable, the identity of the provider, the findings, and the diagnosis.

Some insurers authorize reimbursement of services provided by unlicensed individuals who provide treatment under the direct supervision of a licensed clinician. Other insurers do not allow this and only cover services provided directly by licensed clinicians. This situation is frequently relevant in settings where unlicensed clinicians are receiving supervision from a licensed clinician while gaining experience for licensure. In most instances, these individuals are not eligible for insurance reimbursement. Potential limits to coverage should always be clarified in advance, and all services should be billed accurately. It would be both unethical and illegal to bill for services provided by a supervisee as though they were provided by the licensed supervising clinician.

Not all fraudulent billing is the result of greed or deceit. At times, busy clinicians may make billing errors as the result of carelessness, insufficient oversight of administrative employees, or lack of knowledge of appropriate billing practices.

CARELESSNESS

Fraudulent billing may result from sloppy bookkeeping and record keeping. A busy clinician may see so many clients each day that time is not taken to document the services provided accurately and in a timely manner. Even waiting until the close of business to document the services provided throughout the day may not meet the ethical standards of the mental health professions. It is easy to forget how much time was spent with each client, what services were specifically provided, and what outcomes were achieved. Waiting until the end of the week to do one's clinical documentation would likely result in even more inaccurate records.

Standard 6.01, Documentation of Professional and Scientific Work and Maintenance of Records, of the APA (2010a) Ethics Code, states in part that "Psychologists create . . . records and data relating to their professional and scientific work in order to . . . (4) ensure accuracy of billing and payments, and (5) ensure compliance with law." Thus, it is important that all records be developed in a timely manner as close to the time the service is provided as possible to help ensure their accuracy. Furthermore, records should include sufficient detail, clearly detailing all services provided, so that billing may be done accurately.

INSUFFICIENT OVERSIGHT OF EMPLOYEES

A naive clinician may assume that those he or she supervises clinically or administratively will know all that the clinician knows, will fulfill all obligations the clinician does, and are as timely and meticulous as the clinician. It is essential that clinicians not only ensure their own knowledge of and compliance with ethics, law, and regulations, but also train their subordinates in each of these areas, review changes and updates to these requirements periodically, and provide sufficient oversight and administrative supervision to ensure compliance (M. A. Fisher, 2009). Furthermore, clinicians should never delegate tasks to subordinates that these individuals are not competent to carry out or have not been trained to do. For example, Standard 2.05, Delegation of Work to Others, of the APA (2010a) Ethics Code requires that psychologists "authorize only those responsibilities that such persons can be expected to perform competently on the basis of their education, training, or experience, either independently or with the level of supervision being provided." This standard also requires that psychologists provide the amount of supervision and oversight necessary to ensure that these duties are carried out competently and effectively.

Clinicians who employ staff to carry out administrative tasks remain responsible for all staff members' activities (Knapp & VandeCreek, 2008). Some clinicians assume total responsibility for the billing and collection of all of their fees. However, it is not unusual to delegate these tasks to employees such as an office manager or secretary or to contract this function out to a professional billing service. In some instances, we know that the billing and collecting is delegated to the spouse of the private practitioner. Although each of these individuals or companies may be qualified to do ethical billing and collecting, the clinician still retains responsibility for the actions taken on his or her behalf.

It is recommended that employees undergo periodic training and that a written agreement between clinicians and staff members be used. In keeping with Standard 2.05, Delegation of Work to Others, of the APA (2010a) Ethics Code, it is important to ensure that staff receives the appropriate training to perform these tasks effectively before delegating to them. Additionally, staff must receive sufficient supervision and oversight from the clinician, keeping in mind that the clinician bears the ultimate responsibility for all actions by supervisees and employees (Barnett, Cornish, Goodyear, & Lichtenberg, 2007).

LACK OF KNOWLEDGE

Each of the mental health professions' ethics codes requires that their members be knowledgeable about the content and implications of their ethics codes. Lack of awareness of these standards is not seen as a justification for, or defense against, unethical behavior. For example, in the Counselors' Code of Ethics (American Counseling Association, 2005), Standard C.1, Knowledge of Standards, states that "counselors have a responsibility to read, understand, and follow the *ACA Code of Ethics* and adhere to applicable laws and regulations" (p. 9).

In today's practice environment, clinicians must be knowledgeable about billing and collection practices in addition to those relevant to their clinical competence with clients. Clinicians will need to be knowledgeable about state and federal laws relevant to their practice, such as the Health Insurance Portability and Accountability Act; Medicare and Medicaid laws; and regulations related to workers compensation, Social Security disability, and vocational rehabilitation. Full awareness of contractual obligations under insurance and managed care agreements is essential. Knowledge of ethical standards and the specifics of one's licensing law and other state laws relevant to clinicians is also essential; this includes record-keeping standards, duty to warn or duty to protect, procedures for involuntary hospitalization, and reporting of child or elder abuse.

Naiveté or lack of awareness of relevant ethical standards, laws, and regulations is not considered a mitigating factor when fraudulent billing occurs. For example, a clinician may not be familiar with Current Procedural Terminology (CPT) codes, and this may result in billing for services that were not actually provided. Clinicians may provide 20-minute brief consultations to clients throughout the day. However, not knowing the different CPT codes, they may bill each as a "psychotherapy session" because that is what they felt they were providing. The CPT code for a 45- to 50-minute psychotherapy session is 90806, but the CPT code for a 20- to 30-minute session is 90804. Billing 20-minute sessions as though they were 50-minute sessions (even if not done with malicious intent) would likely result in charges of insurance fraud, bringing significant legal and ethical consequences. A routine audit of the clinician's billing practices would indicate the clinician billing for three 50-minute sessions per hour, something impossible for a single person to do.

Clinicians should also be aware of differences when billing for inpatient versus outpatient treatment services, home visits, and services not provided in person such as over the telephone or through the Internet. Purchasing CPT manuals so that clinicians have accurate CPT codes for their billing is essential so that careless errors are not made.

If a clinician is found guilty of fraudulent billing, regardless of the presence or absence of intent, there can be significant fines and financial penalties, along with the potential to lose one's license to practice, and possibly even incarceration. Thus, such issues should be taken seriously and a preventive approach to accurate billing should be taken. Furthermore, as has been emphasized, this applies both to the actions of clinicians themselves and those of all individuals whom they supervise and employ.

The Most Common Types of Ethical Dilemmas Faced

Clinicians may engage in a wide range of unethical or illegal behaviors relevant to fees, financial arrangements, billing, and collections. For example, in a sample of psychotherapists, Pope, Tabachnick, and Keith-Spiegel (1987) found that 26.5% of those surveyed acknowledged "altering an insurance diagnosis to meet insurance criteria" (p. 80) rarely, and 35.1% acknowledged doing this more frequently, even though more than one third of those surveyed acknowledged that they viewed this behavior as unethical.

In addition to possibly engaging in clear ethical or legal violations, clinicians may engage in behavior that although not necessarily unethical or illegal nonetheless goes against the clinician's personal values. For example, in the Pope et al. (1987) survey, 49.3% of participants used a collection agency at least rarely in an attempt to collect overdue fees, even though approximately 95% of participants viewed this behavior as unethical. Similarly, although approximately one third of those surveyed acknowledged filing a lawsuit to collect fees owed by clients, approximately 90% of those surveyed viewed this behavior as unethical. Despite these practitioners' views of what is ethical or unethical, it should be pointed out that the use of a collections agency or small claims court to collect fees owed to the professional may be done ethically if it is in accordance with professional ethics codes. To ensure ethical practice, professionals must use a comprehensive informed-consent procedure at the outset of the professional relationship that specifically articulates the potential for use of these procedures should fees not be paid as detailed in the financial agreement.

In 1992, Pope and Vetter conducted a national survey of APA members to learn what ethical dilemmas they face in their work. After confidentiality (18%) and blurred, dual, or conflictual relationships (17%), payment sources, plans, settings, and methods (14%) was cited most frequently. Additionally, forensic psychology was reported by 5% of those surveyed and helping the financially stricken was reported by 2% of those surveyed. Examples of ethically troubling incidents reported by respondents include "billing for no-shows, billing family therapy as if it were individual, distorting a patient's condition so that it qualifies for coverage, signing forms for unlicensed staff, and not collecting copayments" (p. 401).

A recent report (APA, 2009) of disciplinary actions by psychology licensing boards between August 1983 and April 2009 provided data on general categories of unethical and/or illegal behaviors that resulted in these disciplinary actions. Of 3,388 total disciplinary actions, 996 were for unprofessional, unethical, or negligent practice; 203 were for improper or inadequate record keeping; 180 were for fraudulent acts; and 155 were for breach of confidentiality. Other disciplinary actions that may have been of relevance to fees, financial arrangements, billing, and collections include inadequate or improper supervision (177) and impairment (133). As the next chapter discusses, each of these causes for disciplinary action and problematic and potentially unethical practices by clinicians can result in sanctions for unethical, illegal, and fraudulent behavior. Each needs to be thoughtfully considered before engaging in them.

Conclusion

Ethical conduct is the result of a thoughtful and deliberative process; it does not occur by accident. A number of important steps can help the clinician to promote ethical practice, both in general and in particular regard to fees, billing, and collections. The following is a list of important considerations for the clinician:

- Be knowledgeable of relevant ethics codes, laws, and regulations relevant to your profession and to the jurisdiction in which you practice.
- Keep current on changes in professional standards and requirements by reading relevant journals, attending continuing education workshops, and participating actively in professional associations.
- Practice ongoing self-care to promote your emotional, physical, spiritual, and relationship wellness.
- When faced with a dilemma and unsure of how to best proceed, consult with a knowledgeable peer or supervisor.
- Always address fees and financial arrangements at the outset of the professional relationship as part of a comprehensive informed-consent process.
- Include all agreed-on fees and billing arrangements in a written financial agreement that is signed by both you and the client.
- Openly discuss and update all agreements when changes occur, whether the changes are brought on by the client (e.g., inability to pay because of loss of one's job) or by you (e.g., a decision to raise your fees in the near future).
- Clarify in advance each individual's financial responsibilities as well as the obligations of insurance companies and managed care organizations.
- Actively ensure that clients understand their obligations from the outset of the professional relationship and again when any changes to the agreement occur.
- Include the possibility of the use of a collection agency or small claims court to collect fees owed in all written agreements. Before implementing such actions, first offer the client the opportunity to make payment. State, and even county and city, laws may dictate specific procedures regarding collection agencies, in addition to existing federal laws.
- Have your financial agreement reviewed by an attorney to ensure its legal appropriateness.
- Ensure understanding of any limits to coverage, reimbursement requirements, and utilization review policies before agreeing to participate in insurance and managed care.

- Clarify with clients the limits of their insurance coverage at the outset of treatment and develop realistic treatment plans that are consistent with these limits.
- Actively advocate for clients through appeals of adverse utilization review decisions, but never modify diagnoses in an effort to obtain authorization for a client's needed treatment.
- Only reduce or waive co-payments on rare occasions, never as a matter of ongoing practice.
- Be educated about insurance and billing matters, understand procedure codes and use them accurately, and ensure that all claims are accurate before submitting them.
- When delegating tasks to others, ensure their competence by training them and adequately overseeing their ongoing activities relevant to fees, billing, and financial arrangements.
- Document all services provided accurately and in a timely manner.
- Develop and maintain accurate financial records in addition to each client's clinical record.
- Participate in ongoing continuing education and professional development activities to remain abreast of changes in ethical standards, regulations, and laws. Ignorance is not bliss, and many commonly occurring problems can be avoided with careful attention to these important sources of information.
- Read all contracts carefully, and consult with an attorney who reviews them for you. When unsure of the appropriateness of a particular action, consult your attorney before taking that action.

Fraud, Abuse, and Case Examples | 8

A s Hannigan (2006) explained, fraud involves billing for services in a manner that seeks higher reimbursement than is appropriate on the basis of the services provided. Fraud is differentiated from abuse in that "fraud implies *intention* to be dishonest" (p. 512), whereas abuse may be due to carelessness or being misinformed about appropriate procedures. Regardless, both fraud and abuse are inappropriate and fall below prevailing professional standards and each profession's expectations of their members.

This chapter discusses the ethical and legal foundations for fraud and abuse, along with case studies demonstrating that fraud and abuse can occur even when the clinician is well intentioned. To avoid these serious lapses, the clinician must adhere to ethical and legal standards.

Ethical Foundations

The American Psychological Association (APA; 2010a) Ethics Code requires in Standard 6.04, Fees and Financial Arrangements, that "psychologists' fee practices are consistent with law" and that "psychologists do not misrepresent their fees." Additionally, Standard 5.01, Avoidance of False or Deceptive Statements, makes it clear that "psychologists do not make false, deceptive, or fraudulent statements concerning . . . their services; . . . their fees" and Standard 6.06, Accuracy in Reports to Payors and Funding Sources, requires that

> in their reports to payors for services or sources of research funding, psychologists take reasonable steps to ensure the accurate reporting of the nature of the service provided or research conducted, the fees, charges, or payments, and where applicable, the identity of the provider, the findings, and the diagnosis.

These specific standards are based on the aspirational Principle C: Integrity in the APA (2010a) Ethics Code, which states that "psychologists seek to promote accuracy, honesty, and truthfulness in the science, teaching, and practice of psychology. In these activities psychologists do not steal, cheat, or engage in fraud, subterfuge, or intentional misrepresentation of fact."

Similar guidance is provided in the ethics codes of the other mental health professions. The Code of Ethics of the American Association for Marriage and Family Therapy (AAMFT; 2001) states in Principle VII, Financial Arrangements, "Marriage and family therapists represent facts truthfully to clients, third party payors, and supervisees regarding services rendered" (para. 67). Standard 5.01, Integrity of the Profession, of the National Association of Social Workers (NASW; 2008) Ethics Code states that "social workers should work toward the maintenance and promotion of high standards of practice" (para. 139). More specifically, Standard 4.04, Dishonesty, Fraud, and Deception, states that "social workers should not participate in, condone, or be associated with dishonesty, fraud, or deception" (para. 129). The American Counseling Association's (ACA; 2005) Code of Ethics requires in Standard C.6.b., Reports to Third Parties, that "counselors are accurate, honest, and objective in reporting their professional activities and judgments to appropriate third parties, including courts, health insurance companies, those who are the recipients of evaluation reports, and others" (p. 10). More generally in Standard C.6.d., Exploitation of Others, it states that "counselors do not exploit others in their professional relationships" (p. 10).

Legal Foundations

Licensing laws for each mental health profession contain provisions similar to those cited from the mental health professions' ethics codes. For example, the licensing law for psychologists in Maryland contains both general and specific standards that speak to these matters (State of Maryland, 1992). In this law, it is specified that psychologists may have their license to practice denied, reprimanded, suspended, or revoked for any of the following violations:

> Practices psychology fraudulently or deceitfully; Submits a false statement to collect a fee; Willfully makes or files a false report or record in the practice of psychology; Behaves immorally in the practice of psychology; Commits an act of unprofessional conduct in the practice of psychology; Does an act that is inconsistent with generally accepted professional standards in the practice of psychology. (para. 1)

Each clinician will find similar legal standards in their own state licensing law. Thus, there are both ethical and legal mandates to prevent the occurrence of fraud and abuse in our professional work.

Understanding Fraud and Abuse

Fraud and abuse pertain to services billed to both government programs and private insurers. In their article about Medicare and Medicaid billing fraud and abuse by psychologists, Gasquoine and Jordan (2009) provided a wealth of valuable information that applies to the billing of professional services. They highlighted that fraud pertains to "cases involving deception that is viewed as intentional (e.g., billing for services not provided, filing false claims)" (p. 280) and that abuse involves "provider practices that result in unnecessary cost to Medicare/Medicaid (e.g., providing services not deemed medically necessary, billing for services provided by unqualified individuals, furnishing erroneous information)" (p. 280). The Centers for Medicare and Medicaid Services (CMS; n.d.) provides the following definitions of these terms:

> Fraud: To purposely bill for services that were never given or to bill for a service that has a higher reimbursement than the service produced. Abuse: Payment for items or services that are billed by mistake by providers, but should not be paid for by Medicare. This is not the same as fraud.

Furthermore, as Hannigan (2006) explained, "These definitions hold true for private insurers as well" (p. 512).

The government has a vested interest in identifying fraud and abuse by all health service providers and facilities. Iglehart (2009) cited data indicating that a conservative estimate is that $60 billion is lost to fraud each year. Because of this, the federal government has allocated significant resources to uncovering fraud and abuse and to recovering this money when possible. Citing data from the Office of the Attorney General of the U.S. Department of Health and Human Services, Gasquoine and Jordan (2009) reported that "in 2006 (the most recent year for which figures are available), the Medicaid program alone recovered more than $1.1 billion in court-ordered restitution, fines, civil settlements, and penalties from 676 successful fraud cases nationwide" (p. 279). It is clear is that the government is serious about fraud and abuse and will actively and aggressively seek restitution when they think it appropriate. It is also important to note that these cases are not limited to physicians but include various types of clinicians as well.

A wide range of professional behaviors fall within the definitions of fraud and abuse. Gasquoine and Jordan (2009, p. 280) provided a detailed list of such activities:

> (a) billing for services not provided; (b) misrepresenting the diagnosis to justify payment; (c) soliciting, offering, or receiving a kickback; (d) unbundling or *exploding* charges (bundled services are supposed to be paid at a group rate); (e) falsifying certificates of medical necessity, plans of treatment, or medical records to justify payment; and (f) billing for a different service than the one provided, known as *upcoding* (Edwards et al., 2003).

Although mental health clinicians may face dilemmas and challenging situations in which how they should proceed may not be clear, specific guidance is readily available to assist us to bill and submit claims ethically and legally. For example, guidance is provided on the CMS website (http://www.cms.hhs.gov). Most professional associations have professional affairs officers who are expert in billing, ethics, and insurance regulations and laws, and these associations and other organizations frequently offer workshops to assist practitioners in this area of practice.

Case Examples and Discussion

JUST TRYING TO HELP

A licensed clinical social worker receives a referral of a couple whose marriage is in great distress. They have been referred by one of the clinician's primary referral sources and are reported to be highly motivated to work with him in treatment. The social worker is a participating provider in their health insurance and is skilled and experienced in clinical work with couples. In reviewing their insurance benefits, the social worker learns that marital or couples psychotherapy is not a covered benefit; only individual psychotherapy is reimbursable. The couple is in great distress and highly motivated for treatment, but they report they cannot afford to pay the full fee for treatment. They report having two children in college, and the wife recently was laid off from her job. The social worker wants to help them and not disappoint his referral source, but decides that he cannot afford to lower his fee. At the couple's request, the social worker lists the husband as the identified client, listing his diagnosis as depression (which is accurate in the social worker's professional opinion), and bills the treatment sessions under Current Procedural Terminology (CPT) code 90806, Individual Psychotherapy, 45 to 50 minutes.

DISCUSSION

Although this social worker should be commended for his great desire to help others and his commitment to ensuring that all those in distress receive needed treatment services, treatment and billing have been done in a fraudulent manner. It is important that the social worker first be familiar with the contract he signed with the insurance company. Failure to be aware of contractual arrangements and the limits of this contract is not a defense against a charge of fraudulent behavior. The social worker violated the terms of the contract and filed claims stating that one service (individual psychotherapy to the husband for his depression) was provided when in fact a different service was provided (marital counseling to the couple). Even if the husband's depression was addressed in the couples counseling sessions, the service provided and billed to the insurance company was not a covered service (couples counseling). Although the social worker's intentions may appear honorable, this is nonetheless a clear case of fraudulent behavior.

THE ILL-INFORMED PSYCHOLOGIST

A licensed psychologist signed a contract to provide mental health services to the residents of a nursing home. The psychologist conducted a no-fee screening of each resident and then provided any requested and needed mental health treatment services after receiving a written order from the facility's physician. She provided both individual and group sessions to the nursing home residents. She provided billing statements to the nursing home's billing department, which then filed the claims with Medicare. As a Medicare provider, the psychologist had agreed to accept the fees paid by Medicare and did not bill the nursing home for any additional fees. Everyone seemed happy with this arrangement, the facility's morale had never been higher, and the residents provided positive feedback on the care they were receiving.

The psychologist and the nursing home's administrator were then shocked when contacted by Medicare and informed that a routine audit of the claims filed revealed a pattern of fraud. The investigation indicated that the psychologist had been billing up to three 90806 45- to 50-minute psychotherapy treatment sessions per hour with up to 26 hours of individual psychotherapy being billed on some days. When questioned, the psychologist reported that she did not know there were different CPT codes for different treatment services; she had been providing 20-minute brief treatment sessions and 90-minute group psychotherapy, yet had been billing as though she was meeting individually with residents for 45 to 50 minutes each time.

DISCUSSION

Knowledge of billing and coding requirements is essential for every mental health clinician. For example, some of the relevant codes for billing the services in the nursing home include the following:

- 90816 Individual psychotherapy 20–30 minutes as an Inpatient
- 90818 Individual medical psychotherapy 45–50 minutes as an Inpatient
- 90853 Group psychotherapy

CPT codes are different for each service provided. There are different codes for inpatient and outpatient services and for individual, family, and group treatment. For appropriately trained psychologists, there are codes for psychological testing and neuropsychological assessment. Failure to become knowledgeable about these codes is not considered an appropriate justification for submitting false claims to collect fees. Mental health clinicians must educate themselves on these procedure codes and ensure that all claims are accurate before submitting them. Even though the nursing home's billing department filed the claims, the psychologist provided the billing staff with the completed claims forms. Her signature on these forms signified that she was certifying that these claims were accurate. Although one could argue whether this psychologist's actions constituted fraud or abuse (because she claimed no intent to defraud the government), she was liable for returning all fees collected plus interest and significant penalties, and then her licensing board was notified that she had been found in violation by Medicare. If ill intent could be proved, she would also be liable for criminal penalties.

HELPING CLIENTS DESPITE THEIR INSURANCE COMPANY

A psychologist conducted an initial assessment of a new client and determined that psychological testing was required. The client appeared to present with symptoms of possible attention-deficit/hyperactivity disorder, but the diagnosis was unclear. The psychologist wanted to understand the client's underlying difficulties better so that the most appropriate treatment plan could be developed. The client's insurance covered up to 50 outpatient psychotherapy sessions per year as well as up to $2,000 of psychological testing per year. The psychologist submitted the required treatment plan to request approval from the insurance company for coverage of 6 hours of psychological testing to be followed by an initial 12 sessions of psychotherapy. The insurer authorized 20 sessions of outpatient psychotherapy but denied the request for psychological testing. The psychologist appealed this decision, but this was denied; the insurer stated that it was not deemed medically necessary. Knowing the client's needs and wanting to provide the best possible care, the psychologist conducted the psychological testing but billed it as psychotherapy sessions because these had been authorized. When the insurer conducted a routine audit of treatment records, the psychologist was found to have engaged in fraudulent behavior, was removed and banned from the insurance network, and was reported to the licensing board and the state's insurance commissioner. The psychologist faced loss of her license, significant fines, and possible jail time. She now had to go through the time-consuming and costly process of defending herself.

DISCUSSION

Many mental health clinicians have experienced significant frustrations with managed care and insurance companies, including difficulties obtaining authorization for coverage of needed services (Murphy, DeBernardo, & Shoemaker, 1998). Often, it may seem that utilization review decisions are fiscally motivated in favor of the insurance company. However, clinicians must work within the system by educating utilization review personnel rather than trying to work around the system. The rationale of the psychologist in this example may have seemed reasonable to her. She had obtained authorization for 20 treatment sessions, she needed to conduct psychological testing to understand the client's treatment needs and develop a more well-informed treatment plan, and she billed the insurance company for the same amount of money for each testing session as she would for a psychotherapy session. In fact, she believed that not only would the client receive better care, it would actually cost the insurance company less in the long run because she would not waste time providing treatment through a hit-or-miss approach. To the psychologist, her rationale was sound.

Unfortunately, despite these good intentions and the rationale she used to convince herself of the appropriateness of her actions, the psychologist still has provided one service and billed for another; she provided a service that was not authorized and submitted false claims to collect fees. Regardless of her intentions or her feeling that this was in the client's best interests, the psychologist engaged in fraudulent behavior. In their "Principles of Private Practice Success" in *Financial Success in Mental Health Practice*, Walfish and Barnett (2008) urged clinicians who participate in managed care plans to accept emotionally the limits of such participation on both income and practice activities. The clinician in this case did not do so and simply explained to the client, "Your insurer has decided this is not medically necessary and therefore will not pay for it." As is, it likely would not be difficult to prove an intent to engage in fraudulent actions because the psychologist was specifically informed that psychological testing was not authorized but provided this service anyway. Furthermore, she used the CPT code of the service that had been authorized, clearly knowing that she wasn't providing that service. Unfortunately, despite her rationale and good intentions, the psychologist faced serious professional and legal consequences as a result of her actions.

DIAGNOSING TO OBTAIN NEEDED SERVICES

A marriage and family therapist was experiencing repeated difficulties with utilization review personnel in trying to obtain authorizations for coverage of needed treatment for his clients. A noticeable pattern was developing in which every initial written request was denied, and he then needed to go through an extensive telephone review to appeal the denial. On appeal, only three outpatient treatment sessions were authorized. This proved both frustrating and time-consuming. The therapist had to argue for every authorization and was repeatedly challenged on why clients needed ongoing counseling rather than referrals to community support groups. The therapist has now conducted an initial session with a client with that same insurance who clearly needs ongoing treatment services. Rather than subject himself to the same irritating—and in his opinion unnecessary—utilization review hassles, the marriage and family therapist submits an initial treatment request for this client and changes the Global Assessment of Functioning Score (GAF) from 70 (some mild symptoms or some difficulty in social, occupational, or school functioning) to a GAF score of 50 (serious symptoms or any serious impairment in social, occupational, or school functioning; *Diagnostic and Statistical Manual of Mental Disorders*, 4th ed., text revision; American Psychiatric Association, 2000). In addition, rather than provide the appropriate diagnosis of 309.0, Adjustment Disorder with Depressed Mood, the therapist listed it as 296.32, Major Depression, Moderate, Recurrent. Later, when the therapist decided that the client needed inpatient treatment to obtain needed services during a time of significant stress in the client's life, he reported that the client was actively suicidal despite knowing that the client only experienced vague suicidal ideation and no intent or plan.

DISCUSSION

As Bilynsky and Vernaglia (1998) highlighted, mental health clinicians may at times claim a more severe diagnosis than is clinically warranted in the hope of obtaining authorization for what they consider to be necessary treatment. Despite his good intentions of ensuring that his client received these services, this marriage and family therapist has intentionally submitted false statements to collect a fee—a clearly fraudulent activity. The therapist knew that the information he provided to the insurance company was not correct but that the treatment provided would be the same regardless of the diagnosis or GAF score. Thus, the client would receive necessary treatment and the therapist would be spared needless hassles and time spent justifying the proposed treatment. However, despite these rationalizations for his behavior, the therapist's actions cannot be justified. Rather than alter the GAF score and diagnosis, the therapist should have engaged in active advocacy—on behalf of counseling clients in general and for this client in particular. In addition to risking great professional and legal consequences, the therapist also is possibly harming the client by submitting the exaggerated diagnosis. Mental health diagnoses submitted to health insurance companies can follow a client, and once in an individual's record they may be difficult to remove. Diagnoses should be given to clients with great care and should be accurate to ensure that clients are receiving appropriate treatment. Altering or exaggerating them in efforts to obtain authorizations is never an acceptable action.

USING ASSISTANTS TO EXPAND ONE'S PRACTICE

A neuropsychologist with a busy assessment and treatment practice was receiving more referrals that she could handle. Rather than decline referrals, she hired two assistants, one for treatment and one to conduct neuropsychological assessments. The neuropsychologist conducted all initial sessions with new clients and then delegated assessment and treatment services to her assistants. The testing assistants administered and scored all tests, drafted a preliminary report for each assessment conducted, and then submitted this to the neuropsychologist. The neuropsychologist then carefully reviewed each report and signed it because she was the supervising clinician. For clients requiring treatment, the neuropsychologist conducted each client's initial assessment, helped to develop his or her treatment plan, and supervised her assistants who provided the treatment.

Insurance claims were billed under 96118, Neuropsychological Testing, Interpretation and Reporting per hour by a psychologist, and 97770, Cognitive Rehabilitation, signed by the neuropsychologist as providing the treatment. When a client received an explanation of benefits form in the mail indicating that the neuropsychologist conducted the neuropsychological testing and the cognitive rehabilitation, the client filed a complaint with the insurance company, the state insurance commissioner's office, and the state licensing board.

DISCUSSION

Delegating to subordinates only those tasks that they are competent to provide and supervising them sufficiently to ensure that professional services are provided competently and ethically is essential for all supervising clinicians. However, even so, it is vital that clinicians bill for these services provided by subordinates accurately and honestly. To bill for services provided by another individual as though they were performed by the neuropsychologist constituted a fraudulent activity. Although providing clinical supervision and reviewing written reports are important activities, they do not replace the need to report accurately who provided each professional service being billed. The neuropsychologist should have billed the neuropsychological testing as 96119, Neuropsychological Testing per hour by a technician, for each hour of assessment conducted by the assistant, and only used the CPT code of 96118 for those assessment services the neuropsychologist actually performed. Although the CPT code of 97770, Cognitive Rehabilitation, is correct, the insurance form needed to indicate that the psychologist had not actually provided the clinical service. This may be of relevance to insurance companies because neuropsychologists and testing technicians typically bill at different rates. To have the service provided by the technician but then to bill at the neuropsychologist's higher rate constitutes a fraudulent activity and is clearly an example of submitting a false statement to collect a fee.

FEES AND REFERRALS

A social worker in a busy practice receives a fee of $200 for every client she refers to a local inpatient substance abuse treatment program who completes at least 1 week of this treatment. Although there are other substance abuse treatment facilities in the local area, the social worker typically refers all clients in need of treatment to this facility. When questioned about this, she reported that this referral pattern is due to the fact that she considers this particular substance abuse treatment program to be the best one in the region. She also has a strong belief that most substance abusers will benefit from the structure of an inpatient treatment program, so in general, all clients with substance abuse difficulties are referred for inpatient treatment.

DISCUSSION

Although this scenario is not relevant to fraud or abuse, it is nonetheless a challenging ethical issue. Even if the treatment facility in question truly is the best one in the region, the fact that the social worker receives a fee solely for making a referral (not for providing actual professional services to the client) creates at least the appearance of a conflict of interest situation. Not only is where clients are referred for treatment at issue, but the fact that clients are generally referred for costly inpatient treatment despite the availability of a wide range of outpatient treatment alternatives and options leaves one wondering what role the referral fees play in the social worker's assessment of each client's treatment needs and the referrals that are made.

Standard 2.06, Referral for Services, of the NASW (2008) Ethics Code states, "Social workers are prohibited from giving or receiving payment for a referral when no professional service is provided by the referring social worker" (para. 83). The intent of this standard is to ensure that the social worker's judgment is not impaired by the promise of a referral fee. Again, even the appearance of a conflict of interest can call into question the social worker's judgment and the appropriateness of the referral. Similar standards are found in each of the other mental health professions' ethics codes. For example, the APA (2010a) Ethics Code in Standard 6.07, Referrals and Fees, requires that

> when psychologists pay, receive payment from, or divide fees with another professional, other than in an employer–employee relationship, the payment to each is based on the services provided (clinical, consultative, administrative, or other) and is not based on the referral itself.

Further, the AAFMT (2001) code states, "Marriage and Family Therapists do not offer or accept kickbacks, rebates, bonuses, or other remuneration for referrals; fee-for-service arrangements are not prohibited" (para. 64).

MISSED APPOINTMENTS AND INSURANCE

A licensed professional counselor in independent practice ensures that all clients know her policy that she charges for all missed appointments and those that are canceled with less than 24 hours' notice. This policy is discussed during the informed-consent process and is printed on the receipt clients receive at the end of each session. When a client has canceled three appointments at the last minute and then rescheduled them because of scheduling conflicts in her busy life, the counselor reminds the client of her late cancelation policy and bills her for these three sessions. The client is upset and states that she cannot afford to continue treatment if she has to pay for them. Wanting to be fair to both of them, the counselor agrees to invoice the insurance company for these sessions, billing them as though they were treatment sessions that actually had been provided (CPT 90806). When the client's insurance benefits for the year are exhausted, the client complains to the insurer that she should have an additional three sessions under her plan. When this is investigated, the three inappropriately billed sessions are discovered. The counselor is charged with insurance fraud and her licensing board is informed of this as well.

DISCUSSION

Although the counselor was attempting to assist her client, she nonetheless was committing insurance fraud. If the client's insurance policy provided coverage for missed or last-minute canceled appointments, they should have been billed as such. However, most insurance policies only provide coverage for services that are actually provided. The counselor should have engaged in ongoing discussions with her client and addressed the issue of financial responsibility the first time an appointment was canceled with inadequate notice. Perhaps the counselor should not have scheduled any additional appointments until the financial matter was resolved. Allowing outstanding debt to build up tends to exacerbate the situation. Submitting a claim for actual treatment sessions that did not occur can never be justified and clearly constitutes insurance fraud.

BALANCE BILLING

A licensed professional counselor who is a participating provider in an insurance plan has seen the fees allowed by the insurer reduced each year. Despite ever-increasing expenses such as rent, utilities, and the like, he has not increased his fees to clients in more than 4 years. However, over this time, the amount he receives from the insurer per session has decreased by 40%. To help make ends meet, the counselor begins billing clients for the difference between the amount charged per session and the amount collected from the insurance company (minus the client's co-payment, of course). He explains this to his clients before enacting this new billing practice, yet after a short time, one of his clients files a complaint, and the counselor find himself under investigation for insurance fraud.

DISCUSSION

The practice the counselor in this example engaged in, known as *balance billing*, is illegal and goes against contractual agreements with insurance companies. When signing contracts with insurance companies, clinicians are agreeing to accept what the insurer determines as their usual customary rate. Although the counselor may have felt that this reimbursement rate was inappropriate, he had signed a contract to accept this amount, and to bill a client for anything more than the agreed-on co-payment violates the contract and constitutes insurance fraud. Regardless of the amount the counselor charges clients, he must accept the co-payment and reimbursement that are specified in his contract with the insurer.

The counselor in this example could have given the insurance company written notice to terminate the contract, as was specified in his contract with the insurer (typically 90 days), and then when the terminated contract was received by the counselor, he would no longer have been bound by the insurance company's reimbursement rates. However, he also would no longer have been a participating provider, clients would have been responsible for his full fee, and they would then have had to accept the reimbursement rate specified in their insurance contract. Of course, if the counselor had taken this option, he would have needed to provide clients with advance notice of this status change and should have offered to assist clients who chose to continue with an in-network provider with the referral process.

BILLING INCORRECTLY BECAUSE OF CARELESSNESS AND SHODDY DOCUMENTATION

A marriage and family therapist with a busy practice keeps receiving new referrals. It is challenging for her to keep up with the workload and pace, but she does not want to disappoint any of her referral sources and wants to assist all those who are in need. Although endeavoring to provide high-quality clinical services, the therapist finds herself falling behind on documentation. In fact, over time, she finds herself documenting her week's treatment sessions over the weekend. She believes she has a good memory but often finds herself struggling to remember the length of treatment sessions, fees charged, and services provided. When completing insurance forms, she does her best, and if unsure, always bills at what she considers the lowest likely fee so as not to overcharge the insurance company. However, when a client challenges a reimbursement check from the insurance company as not being consistent with the actual fee charged, the therapist is charged with insurance fraud.

DISCUSSION

Timely and accurate record keeping is essential for all clinicians. This includes both clinical records and financial records. Trusting one's memory is not recommended and is not consistent with standards in the mental health professions' codes of ethics and licensing laws. Although a busy practice with many billable hours is the goal of any clinician, time must be set aside for ongoing documentation if quality services and accurate billing are to occur. Failing to document services accurately on an ongoing basis will not be seen as justification for fraudulent or abusive billing practices. In fact, the situation described here would likely be seen as abuse even without intent to engage in fraudulent billing; it would still be a violation of law that could bring stiff penalties.

Mistakes sometimes do happen, even for the most diligent and careful clinicians. Insurance companies realize this. However, once a mistake is discovered, it is in the clinician's best interest to admit it and take responsibility promptly. On one occasion, Steve Walfish had several claims to mail to one insurance company. On that day, he was to see a client who had that same insurance. The client had not missed an appointment in the 6 months that he was in psychotherapy, so Steve decided to mail the claim for that day's session in the same envelope with the other claims. As luck would have it, that was the one day that the client woke up ill and canceled the appointment. The claim had already been sent in the mail. Steve could have "let things lie" and just not billed for the next week's session so no extra monies would be obtained from the insurer. However, that would have been fraudulent, so he wrote a letter to the insurer, with a copy to the client, indicating that a mistake had been made in billing and to please not pay on the claim. A copy of this letter (with the client's named changed) appears in Exhibit 8.1. Insurers tend to be forgiving of honest mistakes. If Steve had been audited and it had been seen that he billed for a session that did not take place, the insurer would likely not have been so forgiving.

EXHIBIT 8.1

Sample Letter to Insurance Carrier for Billing Mistake

Steven Walfish, PhD
2004 Cliff Valley Way, Suite 101

Atlanta, Georgia 30329
(404) 728-0728

March 23, 2010

To: Aetna Insurance

From: Steven Walfish, PhD

Re: Mistake in Submission of Claim for Mr. John Q. Public

On March 18, 2010, I was to see Mr. Public for an individual psychotherapy session (CPT Code 90806). However, Mr. Public canceled that session because of illness, and therefore it did not take place.

In preparing my billing for Mr. Public, I inadvertently submitted a claims form for this session. As such, I am requesting that you not pay on this session because it did not take place.

Mr. Public's ID Number is W9876 5432.

I apologize for any inconvenience that this may have caused.

Thank you for your attention to this matter, and if you have any further questions, please do not hesitate to contact me.

Cc: Mr. John Q. Public, 5678 Main Street, Atlanta, GA 30047

Epilogue

n the preceding chapters, we have attempted to integrate the practical steps in billing and collecting with sound ethical reasoning and practices. If these practices are followed, we believe clinicians will optimize their incomes while ensuring that client rights are safeguarded.

In this epilogue, we summarize important steps to follow in the billing and collections process. These steps include what to do before billing, before scheduling the first appointment with a client, during the first session, and after having provided the service.

If you are a provider for an insurance plan or a managed care organization (MCO), before seeing your first client, it is important that you become familiar with the policies and procedures as they relate to authorizations, billing and collecting, and termination of services. It is also important to become aware of any appeals processes that have been set in place. This is your contract with each of the companies, and each may have its own unique guidelines and circumstances. Have in place a systematic and organized billing system, whether this is done with a commercially purchased system or one that is "homemade" using a spreadsheet or word processing system. This is the only way that you will be able to ensure you are paid for services rendered. If an insurer or MCO is involved in a client's care, have a system in place to track and obtain necessary authorizations. If proper authorizations and reauthorizations are not obtained, then no payment is received for the services provided even if they were medically necessary. Finally, set in place a procedure that enables clients to pay for services with a credit card. This will increase your collections and reduce unpaid debt.

If clients are using their insurance to help pay for part or all of their treatment, before the first session, obtain identifying information to verify and authorize benefits. The information needed includes name of the client; name of the insured, if different; client's date of birth; client's home telephone number and address; the member or subscriber identification number; and the name of the employer. Then contact the insurance company to verify that benefits are in effect. Find out the mental health benefits in terms of deductible (and if it has been met), session limitations that may be in effect, co-pay or co-insurance that is due from the client, and lifetime maximum for mental health payments. If necessary, obtain preauthorization from the insurer or MCO. As part of an informed-consent process, communicate the financial responsibilities of the client to pay for their services.

During the first session with the client, review financial policies and client responsibility for payment and answer any questions related to billing and collection of fees. The financial agreement is an essential part of the informed-consent process. In addition, at that time, have the client sign a credit card guarantee allowing you to bill for any unpaid outstanding balances.

After providing services, collect payments due on the date of the session (co-pays for in-network benefits and agreed-on full fee for out-of-network benefits). This will improve cash flow to pay practice expenses and also prevent a balance from building. Record these data in your billing and accounts receivable system. In the case of insurance filings, carefully complete and submit the CMS-1500 Claim Form to the insurance carrier, whether electronically or via the U.S. Postal Service. Some insurance companies will allow you to bill directly on their web portal. After payment is received by the insurance company, carefully review the explanation of benefits when it is received. If anything is incorrect, send a follow-up letter with documentation to the insurer. After payment is received from the insurance company, if services are not paid in full, bill the client directly for any additional monies that may be due (consistent with the limits of the financial agreement you signed with the insurer; do not use balance billing). If necessary, follow-up with the MCO to request any additional sessions that may be necessary beyond those initially authorized.

These steps will not ensure that you collect 100% of the monies that you have billed for the excellent services that you have provided. However, if followed, we believe they will increase your rate of collections and decrease client confusion or unhappiness with your billing and collecting methods.

Appendix A: Sample Financial Agreement

John Q. Public PhD
Licensed Psychologist
1234 Main Street
Atlanta, Georgia 30329

Disclosure Statement and Financial Agreement

Purpose: This document describes Dr. Public's background and training and will serve as an agreement for him to provide psychological services to you. This document also describes Dr. Public's fees, billing process, and issues related to the billing and collection of fees for services provided on my behalf by Dr. Public.

Training: Dr. Public is a licensed Psychologist in the State of Georgia. To qualify for licensing as a psychologist, he passed a national written examination, a written examination regarding the laws and rules of practicing as a psychologist in the state, and an oral exam by two members of the State Licensing Board. He received his PhD in clinical/community psychology from the University of South Florida in 1981. Before moving to Georgia in 2002, he was licensed as a psychologist in Washington State (1992–2002) and Florida (1983–1992).

Services: Dr. Public provides individual and couples psychotherapy and completes psychological evaluations. Psychotherapy sessions are scheduled to last 45 minutes. Psychological evaluations last several hours and consist of two parts: The first is the completion of a series of psychological tests. This process usually takes several hours. Some people complete the task faster, and some people take longer to complete it. After these tests are filled out, an interview is conducted in which Dr. Public will ask me some additional questions, may ask for clarification on the tests that were completed, and then he writes a report summarizing the results of the evaluation.

Confidentiality: All information discussed in the course of the evaluation is strictly confidential. By law, information can only be released with the written consent of the person treated or the person's parents or guardian. However, the law requires the release of confidential information in three situations: suspected child or elder abuse, potential suicidal behavior, or threatened harm to others or property. In the case of violence toward others, Dr. Public has an obligation to warn the party who may be the potential victim of violence. In addition, in certain select circumstances, a court may order the release of records.

The terms of insurance coverage may require that your records be released for review by the insurance company or their managed care company. In the case of managed care, companies routinely request clinical information in their consideration of authorization of payment for further sessions. Clinical information may include session times; type and frequency of treatment; results of tests; and summaries of the following: diagnosis, functional status, the treatment plan, symptoms, prognosis, and progress to date. Health plans are not legally allowed to require the release of "psychotherapy notes," which are my notes about the specific contents of our conversations during psychotherapy sessions. These notes are kept separate from your clinical record and require your explicit authorization for me to release them to anyone else.

Fees: The fee for the initial consultation, usually lasting 50 to 60 minutes, is $175. Fees for ongoing counseling sessions (45 minutes) are $140.

The actual amount owed to Dr. Public may be lower than these fees if Dr. Public is a Participating Provider for your insurance carrier or managed care company. In these cases, Dr. Public has signed a contract with these groups agreeing to provide discounts on his usual and customary fees.

Fees may be paid with cash, check, or credit card (Visa, Mastercard, and Discover only).

Billing Insurance: In some instances, Dr. Public will be considered an In-Network Provider for my insurance carrier, and there are some carriers for which he will be considered an Out-of-Network Provider.

If he is an In-Network Provider, then Dr. Public "accepts my insurance." He has a contracted rate with the insurance carrier. Through this contract, he will bill the insurance carrier to pay its portion of the fee due for his providing services to me. I will not have to pay Dr. Public and wait to be reimbursed by my insurance carrier. In this case, I am only responsible for any deductible that may not have been met and any co-pay that may be due for the services. I understand that these fees are payable on the day of service unless there is an extraordinary circumstance, which I will discuss with Dr. Public. In these cases, he may choose to make alternative arrangements with me for payment.

If he is an Out-Of-Network Provider, then Dr. Public does not accept my insurance. In these cases, I will pay Dr. Public on the day services are provided. Upon request, Dr. Public will provide me with an invoice that I can submit to my insurance carrier in an attempt to be reimbursed for part or all of the fees that I paid to Dr. Public. I understand that these fees are payable on the day of service unless there is an extraordinary circumstance, which I will discuss with Dr. Public. In these cases, he may choose to make alternative arrangements.

Insurance Company Requirements: I understand that when my insurance company or managed care company is authorizing my treatment with Dr. Public, and when I seek to obtain reimbursement from my insurance or managed care company, Dr. Public must provide them with information related to (a) my diagnosis, (b) the dates services were provided, and (c) the type of service that is provided.

I am aware that as part of this agreement to have these companies pay for my care, they have a right to request clinical notes from Dr. Public to authenticate that care was being provided and the nature of that care. They may also request that Dr. Public complete forms or speak with a representative of these companies to request further authorization of my care. During these communications, Dr. Public will be sharing confidential and personal information about me and my care with these companies.

No-Show and Late Cancellation Fees: If an appointment is not canceled 24 hours ahead of the scheduled appointment time, I understand that, unless contractually prohibited by my insurance carrier, Dr. Public will charge the arranged fee for that appointment. I understand that I bear the full cost of "no-shows" or late cancellations and that insurance carriers will not pay this fee because no actual service was delivered. However, because Dr. Public reserved that time specifically for me, I know that I will owe the entire allowed fee for the session, not just my usual co-pay. I also understand that I may leave a message on Dr. Public's voice mail after hours and on weekends if I need to cancel an appointment. Dr. Public will not charge for no-shows or late cancellations in the case of a true emergency (please note that having to work late is not considered a true emergency) or if I or a child I am responsible for is ill, resulting in my being unable to attend the appointment.

Fees for Administrative Services: There may be some circumstances in which I request that Dr. Public complete forms on my behalf. Some examples of these might include Disability Claim forms, Workers Compensation Claim forms, Health or Life Insurance Application forms, or requests for additional sessions from my managed care companies. I understand that Dr. Public will charge me $25 for the completion of these forms if he does them outside of our session time, or there will be no charge if he completes them during our regular session time. Dr. Public will not charge a fee for corresponding with another health care professional about my care.

Unpaid Balances: I understand that payment is expected at the time of each appointment. Dr. Public will not allow a balance to build up to more than $300 except in the case of a life-threatening emergency. If this becomes the case, then discussion should take place with Dr. Public on how to best bring this balance to zero, while taking into consideration my clinical needs.

In the case in which Dr. Public will be submitting bills directly to my insurance carrier, I understand that he may not receive payment as expected. This may be because of unpaid deductibles (some policies have separate deductibles for mental health care) or because the co-pay due was larger than had been expected. In these cases, I am aware that Dr. Public will bill me, and I will be expected to resolve any unpaid balances within 15 days.

Returned Checks: In the event a check is returned for insufficient funds, I will be charged the standard service charges that Dr. Public's bank charges him for the processing of such a check. There will be no additional costs added on by Dr. Public.

Fees for Court-Related Services: On occasion, cases become involved in the court system. Examples include divorce, custody, and personal injury cases, but there are many others. Fees for court-related services are billed at $350 per hour. This includes any additional consultation with my attorney, preparation for deposition, and actual deposition or court testimony (including travel time and waiting time). All fees for court-related services will be expected to be paid in advance.

I have carefully reviewed and understand this financial agreement with Dr. Public. All my questions about it have been answered to my satisfaction by Dr. Public. I agree to comply with this agreement and accept full responsibility for payment for all services provided to me, or on my behalf, by Dr. Public.

Signature: _____ Date: _____

Assignment of Benefits (for Clients Using Their Health Insurance)

I authorize release of medical or other information requested by the insurance companies or other third-party payers listed above to facilitate claims processing.

I authorize payment directly to John Q. Public, PhD.

I permit a copy of this authorization to be used in place of the original.

I understand that I am responsible for my fees.

Signature: _____ Date: _____

Appendix B: Sample Superbill

Jeffrey E. Barnett, PsyD, ABPP
Licensed Psychologist
Board Certification in:
Clinical Psychology and Clinical Child
and Adolescent Psychology

1511 Ritchie Highway, Suite 201
Arnold, MD 21012
Phone: (410) 757-1511

Maryland License Number: 12345
Tax ID Number: 11-1234567
NPI: 1234567890
Fax: (410) 757-4888

CPT Code	Service Provided	Charge
90801	Initial Diagnostic Eval	
90804	Psychotherapy 30 min.	
90806	Psychotherapy 45–50 min.	
90847	Family Therapy 45–50 min.	
90853	Group Therapy	
90808	Psychotherapy 75–90 min.	
96101	Psychological Testing	
	▪ WISC–IV	
	▪ WAIS–IV	
	▪ MMPI–A/MMPI–2	
	▪ WIAT–II	
	▪ Bender Gestalt Test II	
	▪ Trails Test	
	▪ Color Trails 2	
	▪ Gray Oral Reading Tests—4	
	▪ Other	
90889	▪ Written Report	
	▪ Telephone Consultation	
	▪ Expert Legal Testimony	
	▪ Late Cancellation	
	▪ Missed Appointment	
	▪ Consultation	

DX Code:

YOUR NEXT APPT. WILL BE ON:_____

Day   Date   Time

Patient's Name:_____

Date of Service:_____ **Amount Due:**_____

Signature:_____

Note: Each patient is responsible for payment of the charges due at the time of service. Full charge will be made for appointments not cancelled at least 24 hours in advance.

Appendix C: Sample Insurance Claim Form (CMS-1500)

Form from Centers for Medicare and Medicaid Services. Availability information at http://www.cms.gov/. In public domain.

1500

HEALTH INSURANCE CLAIM FORM

APPROVED BY NATIONAL UNIFORM CLAIM COMMITTEE 08/05

PICA | PICA

1. MEDICARE (Medicare #)	MEDICAID (Medicaid #)	TRICARE CHAMPUS (Sponsor's SSN)	CHAMPVA (Member ID#)	GROUP HEALTH PLAN (SSN or ID)	FECA BLK LUNG (SSN)	OTHER (ID)	1a. INSURED'S I.D. NUMBER (For Program in Item 1)
							24683579

2. PATIENT'S NAME (Last Name, First Name, Middle Initial)	3. PATIENT'S BIRTH DATE MM DD YY / SEX	4. INSURED'S NAME (Last Name, First Name, Middle Initial)
Public, John Q.	11 14 68 M [X] F	Public, John Q.

5. PATIENT'S ADDRESS (No., Street)	6. PATIENT RELATIONSHIP TO INSURED	7. INSURED'S ADDRESS (No., Street)
888 Eighth Street	Self [X] Spouse Child Other	888 Eighth Street

CITY	STATE	8. PATIENT STATUS	CITY	STATE
Atlanta	GA	Single Married [X] Other	Atlanta	GA

ZIP CODE	TELEPHONE (Include Area Code)		ZIP CODE	TELEPHONE (Include Area Code)
30306	( )	Employed Full-Time Student [X] Part-Time Student	30306	( )

9. OTHER INSURED'S NAME (Last Name, First Name, Middle Initial)	10. IS PATIENT'S CONDITION RELATED TO:	11. INSURED'S POLICY GROUP OR FECA NUMBER
		4396A

a. OTHER INSURED'S POLICY OR GROUP NUMBER	a. EMPLOYMENT? (Current or Previous) YES [X] NO	a. INSURED'S DATE OF BIRTH MM DD YY / SEX
		11 14 68 M [X] F

b. OTHER INSURED'S DATE OF BIRTH MM DD YY / SEX	b. AUTO ACCIDENT? PLACE (State) YES [X] NO	b. EMPLOYER'S NAME OR SCHOOL NAME
M F		Georgia State University

c. EMPLOYER'S NAME OR SCHOOL NAME	c. OTHER ACCIDENT? YES [X] NO	c. INSURANCE PLAN NAME OR PROGRAM NAME
		Blue Cross PPO

d. INSURANCE PLAN NAME OR PROGRAM NAME	10d. RESERVED FOR LOCAL USE	d. IS THERE ANOTHER HEALTH BENEFIT PLAN? YES [X] NO If yes, return to and complete item 9 a-d.

READ BACK OF FORM BEFORE COMPLETING & SIGNING THIS FORM.

12. PATIENT'S OR AUTHORIZED PERSON'S SIGNATURE I authorize the release of any medical or other information necessary to process this claim. I also request payment of government benefits either to myself or to the party who accepts assignment below.

SIGNED **Signature on File**   DATE **6/22/07**

13. INSURED'S OR AUTHORIZED PERSON'S SIGNATURE I authorize payment of medical benefits to the undersigned physician or supplier for services described below.

SIGNED **Signature on File**

14. DATE OF CURRENT: MM DD YY ILLNESS (First symptom) OR INJURY (Accident) OR PREGNANCY (LMP)	15. IF PATIENT HAS HAD SAME OR SIMILAR ILLNESS. GIVE FIRST DATE MM DD YY	16. DATES PATIENT UNABLE TO WORK IN CURRENT OCCUPATION MM DD YY FROM TO
06 22 07		

17. NAME OF REFERRING PROVIDER OR OTHER SOURCE	17a.	18. HOSPITALIZATION DATES RELATED TO CURRENT SERVICES MM DD YY FROM TO
Jane Doe, MD	17b. NPI	

19. RESERVED FOR LOCAL USE	20. OUTSIDE LAB? YES [X] NO	$ CHARGES

21. DIAGNOSIS OR NATURE OF ILLNESS OR INJURY (Relate Items 1, 2, 3 or 4 to Item 24E by Line)

1. | 300.02   3. |
2. | 4. |

22. MEDICAID RESUBMISSION CODE	ORIGINAL REF. NO.

23. PRIOR AUTHORIZATION NUMBER

24. A. DATE(S) OF SERVICE From MM DD YY	To MM DD YY	B. PLACE OF SERVICE	C. EMG	D. PROCEDURES, SERVICES, OR SUPPLIES (Explain Unusual Circumstances) CPT/HCPCS MODIFIER	E. DIAGNOSIS POINTER	F. $ CHARGES	G. DAYS OR UNITS	H. EPSDT Family Plan	I. ID. QUAL.	J. RENDERING PROVIDER ID. #
1 07 13 07	07 13 07	11		90806	1	140 00	1		NPI	1111122222
2 07 20 07	07 20 07	11		90806	1	140 00	1		NPI	1111122222
3									NPI	
4									NPI	
5									NPI	
6									NPI	

25. FEDERAL TAX I.D. NUMBER	SSN EIN	26. PATIENT'S ACCOUNT NO.	27. ACCEPT ASSIGNMENT? (For govt. claims, see back) [X] YES NO	28. TOTAL CHARGE	29. AMOUNT PAID	30. BALANCE DUE
000000001	[X]			$ 280 00	$ 0 00	$ 280.00

31. SIGNATURE OF PHYSICIAN OR SUPPLIER INCLUDING DEGREES OR CREDENTIALS (I certify that the statements on the reverse apply to this bill and are made a part thereof.)	32. SERVICE FACILITY LOCATION INFORMATION	33. BILLING PROVIDER INFO & PH # (404) 728-0728
STEVEN WALFISH, PHD 7/20/07		Steven Walfish, Ph.D. 2004 Cliff Valley Way, Suite 101 Atlanta, GA 30329
SIGNED DATE	a. NPI b.	a. NPI b.

NUCC Instruction Manual available at: www.nucc.org

APPROVED OMB-0938-0999 FORM CMS-1500 (08/05)

CARRIER

PATIENT AND INSURED INFORMATION

PHYSICIAN OR SUPPLIER INFORMATION

Appendix D: Sample Credit Card Guaranty of Payment

I understand that Dr. Walfish will be billing my insurance company for therapy or evaluation services. I further understand that I am responsible for all reasonable and customary fees that my insurance company does not pay, such as deductibles or co-pays. I also understand that Dr. Walfish is billing my insurance company as a courtesy to me rather than my paying for services upfront and waiting to be reimbursed by my insurance company. I understand that Dr. Walfish will work with me and my insurance company to receive payment from them. For my convenience, he will wait a reasonable amount of time to be reimbursed by my insurance carrier for services delivered. However, sometimes insurance companies do not pay in a timely manner, and sometimes they do not reimburse at the rate that was initially expected. Because of this, I am giving Dr. Walfish permission to charge my credit card for any services that have not been paid by myself or my insurance company within ninety (90) days of billing. If services have not been paid within 60 days, Dr. Walfish will notify me in writing that he has not been paid by my insurance company and that he encourages me to contact the company to get them to pay for the services in a timely manner. I understand that Dr. Walfish uses the credit card company professionalservices.com. On my credit card statement, the charge will appear as if coming from them and not from Dr. Walfish. I understand that this form is valid for 3 years unless I cancel the authorization in writing.

_____

Patient Name

_____

Cardholder Name (if different from the patient)

_____

Cardholder Billing Address

_____

Type of Credit Card (Visa, Mastercard, Discover—Note: American Express Not Accepted)

_____

Credit Card Number

_____

Expiration Date

_____

Signature and Date

References

American Association of Marital and Family Therapy. (2001). *AAMFT code of ethics*. Retrieved from http://www.aamft.org/resources/lrm_plan/Ethics/ethicscode2001.asp

American Counseling Association. (2005). *ACA code of ethics*. Retrieved from http://www.counseling.org/Resources/CodeOfEthics/TP/Home/CT2.aspx

American Psychiatric Association. (2000). *Diagnostic and statistical manual of mental disorders* (4th ed., text revision). Washington, DC: Author.

American Psychological Association. (2009, September). Reported disciplinary actions for psychologists. *Monitor on Psychology, 40*(8), 13.

American Psychological Association. (2010a). *Ethical principles of psychologists and code of conduct*. Retrieved from http://www.apa.org/ethics/code/index.aspx

American Psychological Association. (2010b). Guidelines for child custody evaluations in family law proceedings. *American Psychologist, 65*, 863–867. doi:10.1037/a0021250

Angerer, J. M. (2003). Job burnout. *Journal of Employment Counseling, 40*, 98–107.

Babcock, L., & Lashever, S. (2003). *Women don't ask: Negotiation and the gender divide*. Princeton, NJ: Princeton University Press.

Barnett, J. E. (2007). Impaired professionals: Distress, professional impairment, self-care, and psychological wellness. In M. Hersen & A. M. Gross (Eds.), *Handbook of clinical psychology* (Vol. 1, pp. 857–884). New York, NY: Wiley.

Barnett, J. E. (2010). Adolescent and (vs.) parent: Clinical, ethical, and legal issues for practitioners. *The Independent Practitioner, 30,* 77–80.

Barnett, J. E., Cornish, J. E., Goodyear, R. K., & Lichtenberg, J. W. (2007). Commentaries on the ethical and effective practice of clinical supervision. *Professional Psychology: Research and Practice, 38,* 268–275. doi:10.1037/0735-7028.38.3.268

Barnett, J. E., & Hillard, D. (2001). Psychologist distress and impairment: The availability, nature, and use of colleague assistance programs for psychologists. *Professional Psychology: Research and Practice, 32,* 205–210. doi:10.1037/0735-7028.32.2.205

Barnett, J. E., Wise, E. H., Johnson-Greene, D., & Buckey, S. F. (2007). Informed consent: Too much of a good thing? Or not enough? *Professional Psychology: Research and Practice, 38,* 179–186. doi:10.1037/0735-7028.38.2.179

Beahrs, J. O., & Gutheil, T. G. (2001). Informed consent in psychotherapy. *The American Journal of Psychiatry, 158,* 4–10. doi:10.1176/appi.ajp.158.1.4

Beauchamp, T. L., & Childress, J. F. (1994). *Principles of biomedical ethics* (4th ed.). New York: Oxford University Press.

Bennett, B., Bricklin, P., Harris, E., Knapp, S., VandeCreek, L., & Younggren, J. (2006). *Assessing and managing risk in psychological practice: An individualized approach.* Rockville, MD: American Psychological Association Insurance Trust.

Bilynsky, N. S., & Vernaglia, E. R. (1998). The ethical practice of psychology in a managed care framework. *Psychotherapy: Theory, Research, & Practice, 35*(1), 54–68. doi:10.1037/h0087839

Blanchard, E. B., Hickling, E., Taylor, A., Loos, W., & Gerardi, R. (1994). Psychological morbidity associated with motor vehicle accidents. *Behaviour Research and Therapy, 32,* 283–290. doi:10.1016/0005-7967(94)90123-6

Blau, T. (1998). *The psychologist as expert witness* (2nd ed.). New York, NY: Wiley.

Centers for Medicare & Medicaid Services. (n.d.). *Glossary.* Retrieved from http://www.cms.gov/apps/glossary/default.asp?Letter=F&Language=English

Committee on the Revision of the Specialty Guidelines for Forensic Psychologists. (2008). *Specialty guidelines for forensic psychology* (4th draft). Washington, DC: American Psychology–Law Society.

Dolgan, J. (2010). The power of plastic: Why credit cards are vital to private practice success. *The Independent Practitioner, 30,* 18–19.

Edwards, D., Ward-Besser, G., Lasecki, J., Parker, B., Wieduwilt, K., Wu, F., & Morehead, P. (2003). The minimum sum method: A distribution-free sampling procedure for Medicare fraud investigations. *Health Services and Outcomes Research Methodology, 4,* 241–263. doi:10.1007/s10742-005-5559-8

Emerson, R. (2009). *Barron's business law* (5th ed.). Hauppauge, NY: Barron's.

Fernandez, P. (1999). The insurance carriers may not forgive you if you forgive co-payments. *Dynamic Chiropractor, 17.* Retrieved from http://www.dynamicchiropractic.com/mpacms/dc/article.php?id=36094

Fisher, C. B., & Oransky, M. (2008). Informed consent to psychotherapy: Protecting the dignity and respecting the autonomy of patients. *Journal of Clinical Psychology, 64,* 576–588.

Fisher, M. A. (2009). Ethics-based training for nonclinical staff in mental health settings. *Professional Psychology: Research and Practice, 40,* 459–466. doi:10.1037/a0016642

Gasquoine, P. G., & Jordan, T. L. (2009). Medicare/Medicaid billing fraud and abuse by psychologists. *Professional Psychology: Research and Practice, 40,* 279–283. doi:10.1037/a0013645

Gelso, C., & Hayes, J. (2001). Countertransference management. *Psychotherapy Theory, Research, Practice, Training, 38,* 418–422. doi:10.1037/0033-3204.38.4.418

Gresham, M. (2009). Ethics and fees in practice. *In Practice, 29,* 100–101.

Grodzki, L. (2004). Making peace with money: The social worker as entrepreneur. *Social Work Today, 4,* 18–20.

Hagen, M. (1997). *Whores of the court: The fraud of psychiatric testimony and the rape of American justice.* New York, NY: HarperCollins.

Hannigan, N. S. (2006). Blowing the whistle on healthcare fraud: Should I? *Journal of the American Academy of Nurse Practitioners, 18,* 512–517.

Hayes, J. (2004). The inner world of the psychotherapist: A program of research on countertransference. *Psychotherapy Research, 14,* 21–36. doi:10.1093/ptr/kph002

Herron, W. (1995). Visible and invisible psychotherapy fees. *Psychotherapy in Private Practice, 14,* 7–17.

Hess, A. K. (1998). Accepting forensic case referrals: Ethical and professional considerations. *Professional Psychology: Research and Practice, 29,* 109–114. doi:10.1037/0735-7028.29.2.109

Hess, A. K. (2006a). Serving as an expert witness. In I. Weiner & A. K. Hess (Eds.), *The handbook of forensic psychology* (3rd ed., pp. 652–697). New York, NY: Wiley.

Hess, A. K. (2006b). Defining forensic psychology. In I. Weiner & A. K. Hess (Eds.), *The handbook of forensic psychology* (3rd ed., pp. 28–58). New York, NY: Wiley.

Hunt, H. (2005). *Essentials of private practice: Streamlining costs, procedures, and policies for less stress.* New York, NY: Norton.

Hunt, H. (2006). Collecting fees right from the start. *The Independent Practitioner, 26,* 206–207.

Iglehart, J. K. (2009). Finding money for health care reform: Rooting out fraud, waste and abuse. *The New England Journal of Medicine, 361,* 229–231. doi:10.1056/NEJMp0904854

Kielbasa, A. M., Pomerantz, A., Krohn, E., & Sullivan, B. (2004). How does client method of payment influence psychologist's diagnostic decisions. *Ethics & Behavior, 14,* 187–195. doi:10.1207/s15327019eb1402_6

Kitchener, K. S. (1984). Intuition, critical evaluation and ethics principles: The foundation for ethical decisions in counseling psychology. *The Counseling Psychologist, 12,* 43–55. doi:10.1177/0011000084123005

Knapp, S., & VandeCreek, L. (2001). Ethical issues in personality assessment in forensic psychology. *Journal of Personality Assessment, 77,* 242–254. doi:10.1207/S15327752JPA7702_07

Knapp, S., & VandeCreek, L. (2006). *Practical ethics for psychologists: A positive approach.* Washington, DC: American Psychological Association. doi:10.1037/11331-000

Knapp, S., & VandeCreek, L. (2008). The ethics of advertising, billing, and finances in psychotherapy. *Journal of Clinical Psychology, 64,* 613–625.

LaFortune, K., & Carpenter, B. (1998). Custody evaluations: A survey of mental health professionals. *Behavioral Sciences & the Law, 16,* 207–224. doi:10.1002/(SICI)1099-0798(199821)16:2<207::AID-BSL 303>3.0.CO;2-P

Lanza, M. (2001). Setting fees: The conscious and unconscious meanings of money. *Psychiatric Annals, 37,* 69–72.

Lasky, E. (1984). Psychoanalysts' and psychotherapists' conflicts about setting fees. *Psychoanalytic Psychology, 1,* 289–300. doi:10.1037/0736-9735.1.4.289

Le, J., & Walfish, S. (2007) *Clinical practice strategies outside the realm of managed care: A follow-up study.* Paper presented at the annual meeting of the American Psychological Association, San Francisco, CA.

Mart, E. (2006). *Getting started in forensic psychology practice.* New York, NY: Wiley.

Melton, G., Petrila, J., Poythress, N., & Slobogin, C. (1997). *Psychological evaluation for the courts: A handbook for mental health professionals and lawyers* (2nd ed.). New York, NY: Guilford Press.

Murphy, M. J., DeBernardo, C. R., & Shoemaker, W. E. (1998). Impact of managed care on independent practice and professional ethics: A survey of independent practitioner. *Professional Psychology: Research and Practice, 29,* 43–51. doi:10.1037/0735-7028.29.1.43

National Association of Social Workers. (1999). *NASW code of ethics.* Retrieved from http://www.socialworkers.org/pubs/code/default.asp

National Association of Social Workers. (2008). *The code of ethics of the National Association of Social Workers.* Retrieved from http://www.naswdc.org/pubs/code/code.asp

Newlin, C., Adolph, J., & Kreber, L. (2004). Factors that influence fee setting by male and female psychologists. *Professional Psychology: Research and Practice, 35,* 548–552. doi:10.1037/0735-7028.35.5.548

Norcross, J. C., & Guy, J. D. (2007). *Leaving it at the office: A guide to psychotherapist self-care.* New York, NY: Guilford Press.

O'Connor, M. F. (2001). On the etiology and effective management of professional distress and impairment among psychologists. *Professional Psychology: Research and Practice, 32,* 345–350. doi:10.1037/0735-7028.32.4.345

Pomerantz, A. M. (2005). Increasingly informed consent: Discussing distinct aspects of psychotherapy at different points in time. *Ethics & Behavior, 15,* 351–360. doi:10.1207/s15327019eb1504_6

Pomerantz, A. M., & Segrist, D. (2006). The influence of payment method on psychologists' diagnostic decisions regarding minimally impaired clients. *Ethics & Behavior, 16,* 253–263. doi:10.1207/s15327019eb1603_5

Pope, K. S., Tabachnick, B. G., & Keith-Spiegel, P. (1987). Ethics of practice: The beliefs and behaviors of psychologists as therapists. *American Psychologist, 42,* 993–1006. doi:10.1037/0003-066X.42.11.993

Pope, K. S., & Vetter, V. A. (1992). Ethical dilemmas encountered by members of the American Psychological Association: A national survey. *American Psychologist, 47,* 397–411. doi:10.1037/0003-066X.47.3.397

Rodino, E. (2005). It's about you: Money and your psychodynamics. In J. E. Barnett & M. Gallardo (Eds.), *Handbook for success in independent practice* (pp. 54–58). Phoenix, AZ: Psychologists in Independent Practice.

Rupert, P. A., & Baird, K. A. (2004). Managed care and the independent practice of psychology. *Professional Psychology: Research and Practice, 35,* 185–193. doi:10.1037/0735-7028.35.2.185

Rupert, P. A., Stevanovic, P., & Hunley, H. A. (2009). Work–family conflict and burnout among practicing psychologists. *Professional Psychology: Research and Practice, 40,* 54–61. doi:10.1037/a0012538

Shapiro, E. L., & Ginzberg, R. (2006). Buried treasure: Money, ethics, and countertransference in group therapy. *International Journal of Group Psychotherapy, 56,* 477–494. doi:10.1521/ijgp.2006.56.4.477

Sharfstein, S. S., Towery, O. B., & Milowe, I. D. (1980). Accuracy of diagnostic information submitted to an insurance company. *The American Journal of Psychiatry, 137,* 70–73.

Shinn, M., Rosario, M., Morch, H., & Chestnut, D. E. (1984). Coping with job stress and burnout in the human services. *Journal of Personality and Social Psychology, 46,* 864–876. doi:10.1037/0022-3514.46.4.864

Sitkowski, S. & Herron, W. (1991). Attitudes of therapists and their patients toward money. *Psychotherapy in Private Practice, 8,* 27–37.

Snyder, T. A., & Barnett, J. E. (2006). Informed consent and the psycho-therapy process. *Psychotherapy Bulletin, 41,* 37–42.

Sommers, E. (2000). Payment for missed sessions: Policy, countertrans-ference and other challenges. *Women & Therapy, 22,* 51–68. doi:10.1300/J015v22n03_06

State of Maryland. (1992). *Health Occupations Article, Title 18: Psychologists, Subtitle 3: Licensing.* Retrieved from http://www.michie.com/maryland/lpExt.dll?f=templates&eMail=Y&fn=main-h.htm&cp=mdcode/14c9e

Sullivan, T., Martin, W. L., & Handelsman, M. M. (1993). Practical benefits of an informed consent procedure: An empirical investigation. *Professional Psychology: Research and Practice, 24,* 160–163. doi:10.1037/0735-7028.24.2.160

U.S. Department of Health and Human Services. (1994, December 2). *Publication of OIG special fraud alerts.* Retrieved from http://oig.hhs.gov/fraud/docs/alertsandbulletins/121994.html

Vasquez, M. J. T., Bingham, R. P., & Barnett, J. E. (2008). Psychotherapy termination: Clinical and ethical responsibilities. *Journal of Clinical Psychology, 64,* 653–665.

Walfish, S. (2001, August). *Clinical practice strategies outside the realm of managed care.* Paper presented at the annual meeting of the American Psychological Association, San Francisco, CA.

Walfish, S. (2006). Conducting personal injury evaluations. In I. Weiner & A. K. Hess (Eds.), *Handbook of forensic psychology* (3rd ed., pp. 124–139). New York, NY: Wiley.

Walfish, S. (2010). *Earning a living outside of managed care: 50 ways to expand your practice.* Washington, DC: American Psychological Association. doi:10.1037/12138-000

Walfish, S., & Barnett, J. E. (2008). *Financial success in mental health practice: Essential tools and strategies for practitioners.* Washington, DC: American Psychological Association.

Woody, R. H. (1994). Payment for forensic psychology. *Florida Psychologist, 44,* 18–19.

Woody, R. H. (1998). Seven ways to incur the wrath of an attorney. *Florida Psychologist, 49,* 10–12.

Woody, R. H. (in press). Letters of protection: Ethical and legal financial considerations for forensic psychologists. *Journal of Forensic Psychology Practice.*

Younggren, J. N., & Gottlieb, M. C. (2008). Termination and abandon-ment: History, risk, and risk management. *Professional Psychology: Research and Practice, 39,* 498–504. doi:10.1037/0735-7028.39.5.498

Zuckerman, E. (2008). *The paper office* (4th ed.). New York, NY: Guilford Press.

Zur, O. (2007). *Boundaries in psychotherapy: Ethical and clinical explorations.* Washington, DC: American Psychological Association. doi:10.1037/11563-000

Index

About the Authors

Jeffrey E. Barnett, PsyD, ABPP, is a professor in the Department of Psychology at Loyola University Maryland and a licensed psychologist who has been in practice for over 25 years. He is a diplomate of the American Board of Professional Psychology (ABPP) in both clinical psychology and clinical child and adolescent psychology. He also is a distinguished practitioner of psychology in the National Academies of Practice. He is a past chair of the American Psychological Association (APA) Ethics Committee and currently serves on the ABPP Ethics Committee and the Maryland Board of Examiners of Psychologists. Dr. Barnett has also served in numerous leadership positions within the profession of psychology, including president of the Maryland Psychological Association and president of three divisions of the APA (Psychotherapy; Independent Practice; and State, Provincial, and Territorial Psychological Association Affairs). In 2009, he received the APA Award for Distinguished Professional Contributions to the Independent Practice of Psychology, and in 2010, he received the Award for Distinguished Contributions to Psychotherapy and Psychology from the APA Division of Psychotherapy.

Dr. Barnett is a frequent author and presenter on ethics, legal, and professional practice issues, including the business of practice. His recent books include *Financial Success in Mental*

Health Practice: Essential Tools and Strategies for Practitioners, Ethics Desk Reference for Psychologists, and *Ethics Desk Reference for Counselors.* He is an associate editor of the APA journal *Professional Psychology: Research and Practice,* as well as the editor of its "Focus on Ethics" feature.

Steven Walfish, PhD, is a licensed psychologist and has been in independent practice in Atlanta since 2002. He received his PhD in clinical–community psychology from the University of South Florida in 1981. He has previously been in independent practice in Tampa, Florida, and in Edmonds and Everett, Washington. He is the editor of *Independent Practitioner* and has served on the editorial boards of several journals. He has published in the areas of substance abuse, weight loss surgery, and professional training and practice. He is currently a clinical assistant professor in the Department of Psychiatry and Behavioral Sciences at Emory University School of Medicine, where he supervises postdoctoral fellows.

Dr. Walfish has received the Award for Outstanding Research in Consulting Psychology from the American Psychological Association (APA) Division of Consulting Psychology, the Walter Barton Award for Outstanding Research in Mental Health Administration from the American College of Mental Health Administration, and the Award for Mentoring from the APA Division of Independent Practice. In 2010, he was elected a fellow of the APA.

His other published books include *Succeeding in Graduate School: The Career Guide for Psychology Students, Financial Success in Mental Health Practice: Essential Tools and Strategies for Practitioners,* and *Earning a Living Outside of Managed Mental Health Care: 50 Ways to Expand Your Practice.*